REALLY TRYING

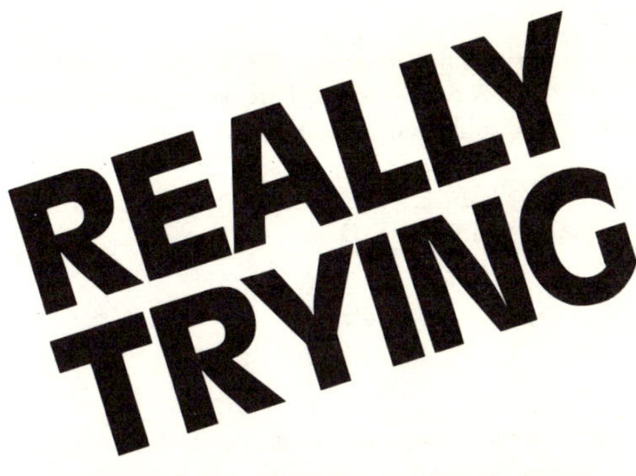

A Career Guide for the Health Services Manager

Anthony R. Kovner

AUPHA Press

Ann Arbor, Michigan

Washington, D.C.

1984

Library of Congress Cataloging in Publication Data
Kovner, Anthony R.
  Really trying.

  Bibliography: p.
  Includes index.
  1. Health services administration—Vocational guidance. I. Title. [DNLM: 1. Health services—Organization and administration. 2. Hospital administration. 3. Health facility administrators. 4. Vocational guidance. WX 155 K88r]
RA440.9.K68   1983   362.1'068   83-24327
ISBN 0-914904-94-9

AUPHA Press is an imprint of Health Administration Press.

Health Administration Press
School of Public Health
The University of Michigan
1021 East Huron
Ann Arbor, Michigan 48109
(313) 764-1380

Association of University Programs
  in Health Administration
1911 North Fort Myer Drive,
  Suite 503
Arlington, Virginia 22209
(703) 524-5500

FOR CHRIS
who was there with me

Contents

PART ONE: THE VIEW FROM ABOVE

PART TWO:
THE VIEW FROM BELOW

PART THREE:
DOCUMENTS FROM THE FIELD

"A wise man makes new mistakes."

Louis Kovner

"The biggest deficiency in my academic training
was that they didn't prepare me for the politics
of a hospital."

Richard Martin

Preface

My purpose is to stimulate self-understanding among persons learning to be health services managers. No one can write down everything such managers do or need to know, nor is this usually attempted—the scope of the field is too broad and change in the field is too rapid.

Some argue that managing health services differs little from managing other types of organizations. Managing health services is like managing food services, managing public health clinics is like managing public housing projects, and managing teaching hospitals is like managing universities. My own view is that managing in health services organizations is distinctive, if not unique. Health services managers can learn more that is helpful by studying health services managing than they can by studying managing in general.

Managing health services organizations is not always what educators and superiors say it is, in part because their interests differ from those of students and subordinates. Educators want to teach students what they know. Superiors want subordinates to do what they say. Many young people enter the health services field to help others, as well as to help themselves. It is saddening that the frustration of their high aspirations often results in cynicism or passive acceptance of ineffectiveness and inefficiency.

This book is a companion to *Health Services Management: Readings and Commentary* and *Health Services Management: A Book of Cases*, both compiled and edited in conjunction with Duncan Neuhauser. The emphasis is on health services managers' managing themselves and those with whom they work, and on their working with physicians. I have chosen to focus on the art and politics rather than on the science of health services management.

This is not a textbook detailing the anatomy of hospital departments and functions. It is not a how-to manual on managing a specific type of health services organization, nor is it a scholarly review or study of theories of health services management. I am not testing a set of hypotheses on organizational theory as applied to health services organizations. Rather, from my perspective of 20 years' experience as a health services manager and educator, I am presenting a view of health services managers really trying to produce results—and trying to keep employed and healthy in the process.

Really Trying is divided into three parts. Part One, The View From Above, is an impersonal analytical overview of the managerial context in health services organizations. It is divided into four chapters: Health Services Organizations, Health Services Managers, Managerial Contribution to

Effective Performance in Health Organizations, and Educating Health Services Managers.

Part Two, The View From Below, takes a more personal form of address as career and on-the-job counselling is emphasized. Part Two is divided into four chapters: Finding Your Niche, Managing Yourself, Managing Your Team, and Working With Physicians.

Part Three, Documents From the Field, mixes maxims, memos, and an interview to particularize and deepen the topics which are presented and analyzed in Part Two. Part Three is divided into three chapters: Maxims for Managers, An Interview with a Hospital Administrator, and Documents from an Administrator's files.

Acknowledgments

It has taken four years to complete this book, during which time I was primarily involved in other activities.

Irene Rosenzweig and Elizabeth Prielozny provided excellent secretarial support through seemingly interminable drafts (before word processing).

I am grateful for the comments and suggestions of the individuals who read various parts of the draft: Martin Chin, John Griffith, Christine Kovner, Susan Sargent, and Norman Urmy, and to Blair Potter, for her invaluable editing of my manuscript.

Tony Kovner

Part One

The View from Above

Your mission, should you choose to accept it, is to take over the management of a large traditional health care delivery system. Your goal for the organization is to maximize the quantity and quality of life for a defined population and with a fixed budget.

Duncan Neuhauser

With relief, we can go back to our present health nonsystem, whose goals are to hustle money wherever it can be found by finagling the reimbursement formulae; where the senior doctors do as they please, and the house staff can run amok with empty order pages in the medical charts; where the goal is to do something for any patient who asks for it, and to ignore those who don't ask.

Duncan Neuhauser

I
Health Services Organizations

"Housed since 1977 in a renovated factory building, the Lutheran Medical Center (LMC) in the Sunset Park section of southwest Brooklyn stands as a testament to the power of ideas over money, of moxie over red tape. To borrow street jargon, it has "finessed" its way through a decade and a half of obstacles, from being a deteriorated institution to being a growing, imaginative one. In the process it helped turn around a lower-class neighborhood long in decline."

Barry Jacobs

"Until 1965, the Davidson Psychiatric Hospital operated in much the same fashion as its sister institutes. It catered to the mentally handicapped in a manner which centered around the dyadic relationship between the physician and patient. Psychiatrists prescribed treatments—usually in the form of drugs, shock therapy and so forth—while the nursing and technical support staff performed the variety of maintenance functions to keep the institution in good running order."

Danny Miller and *Sidney Lee*

This chapter on health services organizations is divided into two sections. The first section deals with the performance requirements of health services organizations. The section is divided into four subparts: goal attainment, system maintenance, adaptive capability, and values integration. In the second section the characteristics of certain health services organizations are specified which bound and define managerial performance.

Organizations can be analyzed in terms of their general performance requirements. What goals do they seek to attain? How do they maintain themselves? How do they adapt to changing circumstances? How do they seek to integrate the values of workers with those of persons who provide the organization with resources and who purchase or regulate its services?

The distinctive characteristics of health services organizations in meeting performance requirements are postulated in table 1. In this chapter I discuss the general tendencies of health services organizations in meeting peformance requirements.

Goal Attainment

The goals or purposes of an organization are defined by those who govern or own the organization. One hospital's primary goal is to generate profits,

Table 1: Characteristics of Health Services Organizations in Meeting Performance Requirements

Performance Requirements	Characteristics of Health Services Organizations
Goal attainment	Difficulty in defining the nature of the service provided Lack of standardized production process Less emphasis on profit and growth
System maintenance	Complicated and indirect reimbursement Highly expensive facilities and technology Labor-intensive services Incentives favoring professional control
Adaptive capability	Varying investment in adaptive capability Varying need for adaptation
Values integration	Heterogeneous labor force Weak integrative mechanisms

given the constraints of obtaining resources and providing services of adequate quality. Another's is to provide high quality care, given the constraints of profits, growth, and medical staff support. There are differences in goals among for-profit, and not-for-profit, and public organizations, and among organizations within each category. There are differences as well in specificity of goals. One hospital's goals may be specified as making a profit, or as making a profit of five percent of sales. Whether a profit of five percent of sales is or is not adequate may be perceived differently by various groups with a stake in the hospital's survival and growth. A profit of five percent of sales may be seen as too small by the hospital's managers and trustees, and too great by its physicians and nurses.

Official and Operative Goals

Official goals are often stated in an organization's articles of incorporation (see figure 1 for an example of a statement of official goals). Such goals may be referred to in the organization's long-range plan and annual report. To some extent, official goals are what officers are willing to disclose publicly.

Figure 1: Philosophy of Service: Community Hospital of East City

In recognition of more than 50 years of existence, The Community Hospital reaffirms its principles and beliefs and makes them known to all who are associated with it in its mission of patient care and community health. The Community Hospital believes in:

Quality Care for All

Good health is necessary to the well-being of every individual, and the Hospital is dedicated, therefore, to providing quality care for all ages, regardless of race or creed and regardless of their circumstances and ability to pay.

Advocacy of Free Enterprise

An atmosphere of free enterprise and individual initiative is the keystone to progress and achievement and offers the best opportunity to render the highest quality health care.

Treatment of the Whole Person

The patient is entitled to more than physical care; his worth as an individual and his spiritual well-being are equally important, and treatment must take into consideration the whole person—his mental and emotional welfare as well as his deep-seated spiritual needs.

Emphasis on the Best

The maximum advantages of modern medicine are possible only through comprehensive health care encompassing the best medical staff working in close harmony with the Hospital, the most highly trained personnel, the most advanced lifesaving equipment, the most up-to-date facilities, and the widest possible range of services.

Consideration for Employees

The loyalty and enthusiasm of its employees are among the Hospital's most valuable assets; realizing this, the Hospital seeks to provide fair compensation, excellent benefits and working conditions, and a chance to advance in accordance with skills and ability.

Stress on Education

Access to educational programs must be perpetuated and expanded to train health personnel for today and for the future, serving the best interests both of the Hospital and the community.

Interest in Research

Research is essential for life and health, and, in support of this belief, the Hospital is constantly trying to implement the latest proven research findings to improve patient care.

Concern with Costs

The patient comes above all and must receive the finest care at the lowest cost consistent with quality. One of the best ways to achieve this is for hospitals to join together for the more efficient management and economic advantages made possible by sharing specialized skills and services.

Figure 1: Continued

Responsibility to the Community

The Hospital must be a responsible community citizen, participating in activities, projects, and organizations that strive to improve the quality of life wherever they exist.

Cooperation with Others

The voluntary health system must be preserved and strengthened; consequently the Hospital devotes its best energies to championing the cause of hospitals throughout the county and in joint planning to avoid duplication and unnecessary expense so that community health needs may be met most effectively and efficiently.

Belief in Excellence

There should be a constant striving toward excellence, and the Hospital seeks to achieve this through dynamic management coupled with a sense of participation and responsibiity by individual employees, aiming at the highest possible standards of performance in all endeavors.

Operative goals include what officers may not be willing to say in public. Shifts in operative goals are reflected in changes in direction and amounts in budgets, or in areas and programs on which owners and top managers spend most of their time.

There may be good reasons for discrepancies between official and operative goals. Certain organizational purposes, such as providing high quality patient care, are difficult to measure or quantify. Seldom is there agreement as to how goals should be specified, not to mention agreement as to priorities among goals. This does not mean that goals are not important or that attempts to specify them cannot be useful; however, beyond general goals, the benefits of specification may not exceed the costs.

Goal Specification

Goal specification involves choosing what the organization will or will not do. (For an example of a hospital's specified goal statement, see figure 2.) Priorities among goals are reflected in decisions about resource allocation. Even if goals are not set formally, decisions about resource allocation are made, but in this case they are made by departments or units rather than by the governing body of the organization. The radiology department will buy a CT scanner, the dietary department will purchase a new meat slicer, the department of nursing will hire ten additional registered nurses or lay off two supervisors. If there are no rules for adjudicating departmental and unit disputes, organizational performance is likely to suffer; that is, it will suffer relative to competitors who can make effective and timely decisions that are perceived as fair by the groups affected.

Figure 2: 1980 Goal Statement: Community Hospital of East City*

Stabilize hospital finances and improve cash flow

Improve board-administration-medical staff communication

Increase hospital involvement in Spanish-speaking community

Fill administrative vacancies and recruit needed medical staff

Increase pediatric and obstetrical inpatient occupancy

Accomplish complete availability of new wing by April 1, 1980 and obtain full hospital accreditation

Establish quality assurance programs for all professional departments

Establish productivity and efficiency goals for all hospital departments

Develop an operational long-range plan, including time and dollar estimates of new programs

Continue to contain increases in hospital costs

*Note: The above goals are only general. Examples of more specific goals would be: for item 5, increase pediatric occupancy to 65 percent and obstetric occupancy to 72 percent; for item 10, contain increase in hospital costs to that of the average annual increase of peer group hospitals in the state.

If goal specification is so important, why do so many health services organizations spend so little time specifying goals, monitoring organizational performance relative to those goals, and redefining their goals in response to changing circumstances? There may be several reasons. Competition may be so weak that goal specification is not necessary for adequate performance. An organization may be too small and uncomplicated to require formal goals specification, or it may not be able to afford the specialized staff or management time needed. Officials in a large organization may not adequately specify goals because they wish to avoid intensifying internal conflict. To the extent that physicians and trustees are not paid by a community hospital, for example, they may prefer unspecified goals that do not commit them to anything. For some organizations, goal specification may jeopardize financial or other support from regulators, donors, or volunteers who disagree with the organization's priorities.

Accountability

Accountability of health services organizations can be evaluated appropriately only, I believe, in terms of specified goals that have been agreed to in advance; this agreement can be reached directly, through negotiations, or indirectly, through shared communications. Otherwise, interested groups are not likely to agree as to what the organization was, is, or should be doing.

For example, it is one thing for an administrator whose hospital is being criticized to say that guaranteeing the access of minority groups to primary care is not the hospital's responsibility. It is another thing to say that this is not the hospital's responsibility if it had been affirmed as such in a goals statement shared by hospital officials with minority group representatives and discussed by both sides before any crisis arose. The minority group representatives may not have been satisfied at those prior meetings when hospital officials explained why access could not be sufficiently assured, but, assuming good faith on both sides, it is more likely that such shared information would lessen conflict between the parties.

At the same time, specifying goals can limit organizational flexibility to initiate, expand, dilute, or close current programs. Goals should change, and the mechanisms for re-specifying them should be identified and shared with parties at interest. Health services organizations cannot provide all services to all people effectively and efficiently. Organizations that attempt to do so tend to lose market share to competitors who have focused their efforts on providing certain services effectively and efficiently.

Health services organizations need to decide where to focus their activities—to the extent that market forces have not already decided for them. Given rising patient and payer expectations, such focusing may be necessary for organizational survival and growth.

Specifying and sharing organizational goals clarifies what an organization stands for, what it is and is not, and what it intends to become. A likely result of such specification and sharing is that organizational decisions will be seen less as the personal, arbitrary preferences of a few physicians and managers and more as joint decisions of managers and parties at interest. This does not mean that all key groups have to participate in all organizational decisions, only that those affected by organizational decisions should understand the reasons for such decisions and, when appropriate, be given the opportunity to participate in making and implementing them.

Specifying and sharing goals may generate the support needed to implement policy effectively. Opposition is likely to be diluted when representatives of all interested parties have participated in the decision-making process. On the other hand, opposition may result in major, valuable changes in the implementation of goals. Specifying and sharing in advance of decision making may also generate enough political opposition to kill a proposed policy. Managers may prefer, however, killing a proposed policy before it has been implemented rather than during or after implementation.

Comparison with Nonhealth Organizations

The goals of health services organizations are often similar to those of other organizations. Managers in hospitals, nursing homes, group practices, and neighborhood health centers, like managers of hotels, universities, and beauty parlors, attempt to increase the number of people using their services and the number of services used by each person.

Health services organizations differ from other organizations in that (1) they have greater difficulty in identifying the nature and benefit of the services they provide; (2) they lack a standardized production process; and (3) they place less emphasis on profit and organizational growth.

Difficulty in Defining Health Services

It is often easier to measure how or whether health services are provided than to specify what they are. A health services manager can, of course, count annual patient days in the hospital or member months in the health maintenance organization (HMO) as easily as a car salesman can count cars sold. But what about less obvious cases? Do health services include a back rub given by a nurse or an aide to a hospital inpatient or outpatient? Do they include a lecture and demonstration to school children about the importance of brushing their teeth?

Health services are generally purchased when "patients" are sick, not when "consumers" are well. Thus, patients tend not to be careful shoppers with regard to price and quality. Rather, they purchase the services of a physician who they think will take good care of them and then leave most decisions about what health services to consume to that physician. This is quite different from the way the same person might buy hotel services or beauty care.

Do hospitals, then, sell services primarily to physicians rather than to customers? In a sense they do, as hospitals attempt to attract physicians rather than customers through the provision of sophisticated equipment and adequate supporting services. Hospitals are paid almost entirely by third-party insurers and by government to provide services to employees and citizens. These large purchasers seldom get involved in the decisions that physicians make regarding which services are to be ordered in what amounts.

Lack of a Standardized Production Process

Physicians differ among themselves as to what acceptable standards of quality are. Thus lay managers cannot specify and enforce appropriate production standards. There is considerable disagreement, for example, regarding what level of infections in a community hospital is tolerable and what kind of sutures should be used in the operating room. Health services cannot be standardized in an HMO or group practice if each physician is allowed to particularize the treatment of each patient. Physicians are given a greater amount of discretion than are most professionals in other types of organizations. This includes discretion about how they spend their time as well as how they treat patients, decisions that have a significant impact on the allocation of organizational resources.

Many health workers with different qualifications are paid at different rates to do similar work. In outpatient mental health facilities, psychiatrists, psychologists, social workers, public health nurses, and a variety of assistants, technicians, and aides provide many similar services. The same is true of pediatricians and nurse practitioners, ophthalmologists and optometrists.

Services, therefore, are generally not provided in a way that is consistent with widely accepted standards of quality control.

Less Emphasis on Profit and Growth

Health services organizations are more often under not-for-profit auspices than under for-profit or governmental control. They are defined more as a public good, and access to them is regarded more as a right than are, for example, automobile ownership and beauty care services. To the extent that tax money is used to pay for health services, there is both a political preference and an economic rationale for limiting operating gains of health services organizations. At the same time, competitive risk is lessened for a limited number of licensed providers. Of course, there is a large and rapidly expanding for-profit sector in the health services industry.

For similar reasons, health services organizations tend to place less emphasis on growth and profits. To the extent that not-for-profit and governmental health services organizations are locally owned, there may be no perceived advantage in extending services to other groups. This is particularly so when the growth capital required to extend services to new users would have to be subsidized by payments from existing users or paid for by temporary inconvenience to or diluted power of existing providers. To the extent that the primary work identification of physicians is not to the organizations in which they work, physicians are less likely to favor growth, unless this will enable otherwise infeasible acquisition of new technology.

Tendencies Rather than Rules

These three characteristics of health services organizations are represented as tendencies rather than genetic properties. Health services such as contraceptives and prescriptions are easily specified. HMOs are chosen directly by consumers in comparison with hospitals, which are chosen indirectly through the choice of a regular attending physician. Health services professionals tend to agree on appropriate treatment for certain problems such as filling of dental cavities or setting of broken arms. In many ways, for-profit health services organizations are like other for-profit organizations, despite the lower specificity of the services being paid for in health and the largely indirect reimbursement for provision of health services.

System Maintenance

Obviously, an organization cannot attain its goals if it cannot survive. Therefore one important organizational performance requirement is effectiveness in the renewal of resources. To what extent does the organization take in more money than it pays out? Are aging plants and deteriorating equipment being replaced at a satisfactory rate? Is the organization in substantial compliance with the rules of external regulatory agencies? Four subsystems of system maintenance are finance, facilities and equipment, human resources, and management.

Financial Subsystem

The constraints on and opportunities for organizational performance are largely determined by the financial subsystem.

Organizations vary in their ability to generate sufficient revenues to offset losses and to maintain adequate flows of cash to meet due expenses. Maintaining adequate cash flow is less of a problem for HMOs, which are paid in advance, than it is for not-for-profit hospitals, which are paid after services are provided. Governmental hospitals have minimal cash flow problems if their budgets are adequate and approval of them is timely. This is often not the case, however.

The financial subsystem includes capital, operating, and cash budgeting; pricing and cost allocation of services; long-range financial planning; and collection policies. Some organizations also have endowments to invest and grants to prepare and administer.

Hospital reimbursement is not easy to understand. Hospitals are reimbursed by commercial insurance companies and by persons who lack insurance (to the extent that they pay) on the basis of charges, which are set above costs. Hospitals are reimbursed by Medicare prospectively on the basis of average length of stay, and by Blue Cross and Medicaid at a level below costs (at least in certain states that regulate hospital rates). For example, in a hospital where the radiology group gets paid a percentage of the hospital's gross radiology revenues, bad debts are 10 percent of inpatient and 35 percent of outpatient revenues, and the proportion of procedures paid by different third-party payers varies by radiological procedure, the pricing and costing of radiological services become problematical and have serious practical consequences for those lacking in sophistication.

Philanthropy

Fund raising may be critical to the survival and growth of many not-for-profit organizations. Often it is only by raising funds additional to those generated by operations that these organizations can initiate and operate new services and programs that may eventually be self-supporting. Fund raising is also important in establishing reserves so an organization can respond adequately to any special opportunity or temporary financial setback or crisis. Many not-for-profit organizations can generate substantial additional funds from those whom they serve. The costs of raising funds can be a high percentage of the monies collected, and not-for-profit organizations have been subject to criticism in this area. Even proportionately high fund-raising costs may be justified, however, if greater funds can be raised in the future while administrative costs remain stable, or if the energies and support generated among those who do the fund raising are essential or desirable in other ways for organizational survival and growth. Such support includes referral of friends or group members as prospective patients, rebuttal of criticism of the organization by regulators, and feedback concerning the perceived quality and adequacy of services.

Prestigious organizations that serve the wealthy may have little difficulty in raising substantial funds from patients and prospective patients. For those organizations that primarily serve the middle class, however, fund raising may prove difficult. Such difficulties may be overcome, in part, when fund-raising activities are organized to meet the wishes of volunteers and when funds are earmarked for specific equipment that is perceived as needed and that is not available locally. Dances, auctions, and fairs are held regularly by various kinds of not-for-profit organizations. Even for-profit and government organizations may be able to organize such events, although this is less likely. An important source of income for some not-for-profit hospitals has been the bequests of former patients and their families.

The importance of philanthropy as a percentage of total new capital investment by health services organizations has fallen since the passage of Medicare and Medicaid. Not-for-profit hospitals have increasingly sought capital financing through the sale of tax-free bonds. Special hospital bonding authorities have been established in many states to help hospitals and other health services organizations gain access to needed capital funds in an efficient and predictable way.

Facilities and Equipment Subsystem

Organizations vary in their ability to generate sufficient capital to replace existing facilities and equipment and to finance new services and equipment. Large for-profit multi-unit health systems have less difficulty because they can raise capital through the sale of stock. Governmental hospitals tend to have greater difficulty in replacing existing facilities because this requires legislative approval and additional taxes.

Human Resources Subsystem

Personnel and labor relations have always been important aspects of system maintenance, particularly in labor-intensive organizations. Many large hospitals are characterized by substantial fragmentation and conflict because work is organized by occupational group rather than by the purpose of a unit or department. Thus many different individuals in different occupations must work together in the same unit providing related services to the same patient. A patient may see more than 50 such individuals in a day in his or her room. Members of over 200 different health occupations must be recruited, trained, and motivated. Hospitals have been characterized by high turnover and by increasing unionization and organizing of professional as well as nonprofessional employees. More and more hospitals are equipping themselves to respond to job action by employees and to union organizing campaigns. Some hospitals have to negotiate conditions of employment with several different unions.

Increasing productivity depends in part upon worker participation in a climate of trust. Personnel (human resources) departments and managers should promote such a climate and encourage such participation. Some of the functions carried out by hospital personnel departments include job analysis and description, job evaluation, wage and salary administration, recruitment, screening and selection, communication to employees, training and development, collective bargaining, and contract administration.

Management Subsystem

A fourth important subsystem of system maintenance is management, which includes governance and support activities.

Governance

The management function in health services organizations is carried out not only by managers, but also by trustees, physicians, and others.

A critical aspect of system maintenance is monitoring and shaping the process of organizational decison making. Organizations vary as to who makes what important decisions and as to perceptions about who should make these decisions. Should decisions on recruitment of hospital attending staff internists be left to the chief of the department of internal medicine, or should these decisions be decided upon by a committee of physicians, managers, and trustees? There may be conflicts of interest in specifying hospital needs for such internists, as administrators wish to fill hospital beds and internists wish to protect their practices from competitors.

Who should decide upon the composition of the board of directors of an HMO? Which interest groups should be represented on the HMO governing board? How should HMO board members be chosen? How should HMO board members be made formally accountable, if at all, to their constituent groups? Typically, governing boards decide upon their own composition; however, in federally approved HMOs, members must occupy one-third of the board positions.

Governing board members may be elected by the board itself or by members of a sponsoring corporation or health plan. Board members may be accountable to the constituent groups who elect them. There may be little need for reporting back to group members as long as there are no major service problems; but if there are such problems or if plan members wish to express their preferences for improving services, elected board members can be expected to be responsive.

A key problem for many health services organizations is the making of timely decisions to enter new markets and to abandon ineffective or inefficient programs. The policymaking process should be reviewed regularly by top management and the governing body for its substantiveness, its inclusiveness, and the speed of the decision-making process.

Support Services

Managerial support services include planning and marketing; community, patient, and public relations; data processing and management information systems; personnel and labor relations; legal services; physical facilities and their maintenance; and compliance with regulations. Each of these is discussed in this chapter. In most health services organizations, managers are seen as being legitimately in charge of these activities. Managers are expected to see that adequate support is provided to physicians, nurses, and others involved in direct patient care.

Each of these managerial support services is sufficiently complex to justify its own textbook. Here, I would like to outline briefly some of the important aspects of several that are common in health services organizations. For a hospital organizational chart that includes most of these support functions, see figure 3.

Community, Patient, and Public Relations. Increasingly, health services organizations are allocating additional resources to, and top managers are becoming more involved in, community, patient, and public relations. This is partly in response to competitive pressures and increasing public expecta-

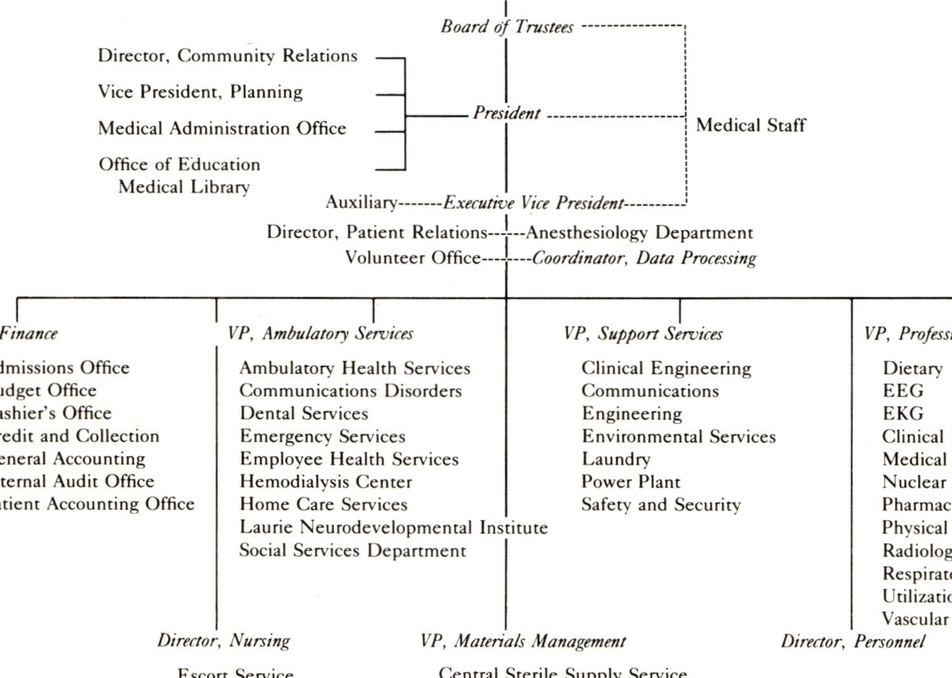

Figure 3: Community Hospital B:
Administrative Organizational Structure

tions. Such activities may also be part of an organization's regular marketing efforts to attract physicians, patients, donors, and political support.

Community relations activities may yield significant benefits. Further, unlike benefits of some other services, these benefits can often be attained primarily through managerial effort rather than through the expenditure of scarce financial or political capital. Representatives of key community groups can be identified and informed. After checking complaints for validity, managers can listen and respond appropriately to group suggestions. Community groups can be advocates for the organization's programs with government agencies that have the power to approve or deny their establishment and continuation. Community relations programs can make potential customers and employees aware of service and employment opportunities provided by the organization.

Volunteers are an important resource in such support activities. They may be one of the key advantages not-for-profit organizations have over governmental and for-profit organizations. Volunteers can replace or supplement full-time staff, enabling organizations to offer services that would otherwise be too expensive. Volunteer services can add significantly to the quality or personal nature of curing and caring. Sitting and talking can provide tremendous comfort to the patient and satisfaction for the volunteer. Volunteers can offer reading materials to inpatients and serve coffee to outpatients; they can conduct patient attitude surveys and provide tours of new facilities for prospective patients. Volunteers can relay back to managers vital information concerning how ambulatory services are being perceived by patients and potential patients. Volunteers can raise funds and may be a source of political support in starting new programs or defending existing ones.

Given the trend toward two-income families, it is becoming increasingly difficult for many health services organizations to recruit effective volunteers. Attention needs to be paid, therefore, to increasing the perceived benefits from or lowering the costs of volunteering. This may be accomplished by providing volunteers with meals and free parking. For their part, volunteers should be expected to meet certain organizational standards, otherwise the costs of using them, particularly in supervisory energies, may exceed the benefits.

Large hospitals frequently employ patient representatives to respond to patient complaints and to better assure patient satisfaction. In some organizations, this function is performed by managers themselves, by direct care providers, and by organizations of patients, such as resident advisory councils in nursing homes.

Public and community relations staff are often organized as one department. Staff in these areas are required to have similar skills. Both functions involve linking knowledge of the total organization with populations targeted for educational and service programs. Public, as opposed to community, relations is often targeted at physicians, nurses, donors, and consumers who can provide the organization with needed resources. Public relations officers typically prepare patient booklets and annual reports, design stationery, arrange for television and radio appearances, and prepare and send out news stories.

It is important for public relations officers to be adequately and promptly informed by managers of organizational policy decisions and their implementation. Otherwise, they cannot reply appropriately to serious criticism of the organization or provide necessary information to potential allies. A public information officer's lack of this kind of knowledge makes the organization look foolish to the media and to the public.

Data Processing and Management Information. Data processing and management information are becoming important support services. If managers are to make effective decisions in the face of increasing competitive pressures, they must be adequately informed and in a timely way. Which of the groups in the population potentially served use and do not use which services? How effective is the organization in delivering effective services to these patients? Accurate information is required to account for organizational expenditures by department or progress in relation to volume of service. Unit performance should be compared with that during past operational periods and with that of comparable departments and programs in other organizations. For an example of a monthly internal management report for an ambulatory care services program see figure 4. Documentation is required in order to validate the identification and to anticipate likely operating problems. Documentation is also necessary in order to influence persons who make policy decisions about whether problems in service, quality, or cost exist or do not exist, and about the extent to which these problems can be alleviated or opportunities grasped to improve service or efficiency.

Three major elements of information systems are the technical, the procedural, and the evaluative. The technical element involves the selection of the appropriate technology for processing data. The requirements of the person-machine system are determined by estimating volume, cost, and reporting standards. The procedural element concerns the development of the necessary recording, summarizing, and disseminating subsystems. Finally, the evaluative element deals with audit, or the methods and administration of the information system.

A revolution in information systems has been occurring in large health services organizations, the results of which have not yet been fully utilized in standardizing the production process. Such standardization is expected to be developed and implemented much more quickly in the next 20 years.

Legal Services. Legal services are provided directly by salaried

Figure 4: Monthly Internal Management Report: Ambulatory Care Services Program C*

Indicator	Jan.	Feb.	Mar.	Apr.	May	June	July	Aug.	Sept.	Oct.	Nov.	Dec.	Total
Summary statistics													
Total encounters													
Total operating costs													
Total collections													
Total cash													
Health center services													
Encounters by type													
medical													
prenatal													
dental													
New patients													
Year-to-date users													
medical													
prenatal													
dental													
New patient ratio													
Encounters per FTE staff													
M.D.													
MLP (Mid-Level Practitioner)													
dentist													
team productivity													
Reception													
No-show rate													
At-visit collection rate													
Financial management													
Break-even ratio													
Charges ratio													
Self-sufficiency ratio[†]													

Collection ratio

Total net charges

Net charges
   Medicaid
   Medicare
   other insurance
   private pay

Total A/R at end of month

A/R by source
   Medicaid/total
   Medicare/total
   other insurance/total
   private pay/total

Months of A/R

A/P at end of month

Operating costs
   salaries
   other

Cost per encounter

Personnel management

FTE staff
   medical
   administrative
   other

Staff turnover rate
   provider
   other

*Reprinted with permission of Aspen Systems Corporation from Owens, Richard et al., "Simplified Manual Systems for Clinical Management: The Internal Management Report," *Journal of Ambulatory Care Management*, Vol. 3, No. 2. May 1980:6.

†The percentage of total costs covered by collections.

attorneys in some large hospitals; smaller organizations often have contracts with outside law firms and professional trade associations. Risk management—that is, preventive programs to avoid malpractice suits—can be viewed as a legal support service. Lawyers can assist hospitals with corporate restructuring, which is the separate incorporation of units or programs of the hospital in order to avoid competitive disadvantages resulting from state regulation or third-party reimbursement. Legal services include developing contractual relationships with other organizations, reviewing service contracts with physicians, advising on purchases of real estate, advising on malpractice and liability claims and on policy concerning hospital rules for the admission of physicians to the medical staff, and advising on patient consent for medical treatment.

Adequate legal counsel may be essential in attempting to obtain fair and appropriate treatment from government regulatory agencies. In the past, many not-for-profit health services organizations, particularly hospitals, obtained legal services at no charge from board members and their firms. Given the increasing amount, complexity, and importance of legal work, however, most of these organizations now must pay for legal services.

Maintenance of Plant and Equipment. Plant operations, biomedical engineering, building maintenance, and allocation of space are other important managerial support functions. Many managers know little about the technical aspects of heating and cooling or about complex diagnostic machinery, yet they may be held responsible in the event of system breakdown, particularly if patients suffer therefrom.

Hospital administrators often find it difficult to allocate space effectively, for political rather than technical reasons. Chairmen of hospital departments sometimes regard their space as inviolable and inadequate for departmental needs and planned programs. In many hospitals, allocation of space is under the control of medical chiefs and department heads rather than top management and is often not allocated efficiently.

Compliance with Regulatory Requirements. Another important managerial support function is ensuring organizational compliance with the rules of national, state, and local regulatory and accrediting agencies. The processes for licensure and accreditation have become increasingly complicated and important for organizational survival. Compliance should be scrutinized closely by top managers, particularly with regard to past violations or recommendations. If such violations or recommendations are not subsequently complied with, third-party payers may withhold reimbursement, and government agencies, licensure. Typically held responsible for compliance, managers can demonstrate expertise in this area and use external demands as a lever to foster organizational change to meet the spirit rather than the letter of certain requirements.

Comparison with Nonhealth Organizations

Some of the distinctive characteristics of health services organizations in system maintenance are complicated and indirect reimbursement, very expensive facilities and technology, labor-intensive services, and incentives favoring professional control.

Complicated and Indirect Reimbursement

Well over 90 percent of Americans have extensive hospital insurance and pay only a small percentage of their hospital bills. Medicare is a federal governmental program that pays for a defined set of benefits, primarily for the elderly. Medicaid is a program funded jointly by federal and state (and sometimes by local) governments; it is designed specifically to serve the poor. Other governmental programs that pay for health services are the Department of Defense, for military workers and their dependents; and Workmen's Compensation, for injuries sustained during or related to employment. Other important third-party payers include over 100 health insurance companies, both mutually owned and commercial, and over 130 not-for-profit plans of Blue Cross (which pays for hospital services) and Blue Shield (which pays for physician services).

Each third-party payer has its own rules and procedures for reimbursement, and these increase the administrative costs of organizations that provide health services. Administrative costs are high compared to similar costs in nonhealth organizations and compared with administrative costs of health services organizations in countries where payment and collection systems are simpler and more unified.

Most hospitals and not-for-profit health services organizations do not raise money for replacing or expanding facilities and programs by allocating a fixed amount of gross revenues or sales to capital projects. These organizations have generally financed their capital improvements through philanthropy, government grant or loan, and, recently, through sales of bonds, with repayment to the bondholders financed largely through reimbursement of depreciation by third-party payers.

Expensive Facilities and Technology

The health services enterprise is large, comprising almost 10 percent of the gross national product (GNP) in 1982, and it is growing rapidly (it comprised less than 4.4 percent of the GNP in 1950). Hospitals represent over 40 percent of expenditures on health services.

The technology of medical care is changing rapidly. New developments over the last 25 years include CT scanning, burn units, renal dialysis, and organ transplants. Equipment is extremely expensive and rapidly changing—hospitals cost over $250,000 per bed, and a CT scanner costs more than $800,000.

Labor-Intensive Services

The health services industry is highly labor-intensive. Over 50 percent of hospital costs are for labor, and the percentage is greater in other health services agencies such as nursing homes or home health agencies.

The two key professional groups within hospitals, physicians and nurses, are relatively independent or becoming more so. Physicians, who largely determine the medical care production process, are only loosely coupled to most hospitals and function largely as independent contractors.

Turnover in hospital nursing has been high. Nursing typically comprises 25 percent of a hospital's budget. Shortages of nurses persist in many hospitals, especially among nurses who work evenings, nights, and weekends. Nursing is in a period of transition. Traditionally, many nurses have withdrawn their services rather than persist in unsuccessfully contesting their working conditions. For a variety of reasons, including the present nursing shortage, the women's movement, and a professionalization movement among nursing leadership, this situation is changing rapidly.

Incentives Favoring Professional Control

Many physicians, nurses, and other professionals have primary commitments to occupational groups that are external to their employing organizations. National organizations such as the American Medical Association or the American Nursing Association often wield considerable influence regarding pay, hours of work, and what professionals will or will not do—and how willingly.

Since the advent and extension of comprehensive health insurance for millions of Americans, many health services organizations have not had to seek new markets, provide services efficiently, or pay much attention to service amenities. Providing health services has been a seller's market, with the supply of hospitals and physicians limited in relation to the demand for services. It is no wonder, then, that managerial attempts to focus on effectiveness and efficiency have been problematic.

Efforts to rationalize production have been frustrated by a lack of scientific knowledge about production efficiency. Agreed-upon output measures are lacking for nursing care, the appropriateness of X rays, the predictable benefits of different diagnostic procedures and therapies, and the appropriate mixes of providers to treat heart disease, cancer, or stroke. Further hampering managers' efforts have been their lesser legitimacy and power relative to that of physicians. This is a result, in part, of the evolution of hospitals, many of which began by providing primarily nursing care, while independent physicians cared for patients at home. Contrast manager-physician relations in the hospital with the more hierarchically determined manager-engineer relations in large manufacturing corporations.

Tendencies Rather than Rules

I am detailing here distinctive characteristics that are not common to all health services organizations. Reimbursement of HMOs is relatively simple, as a per-capita fee is paid in advance each month by the employer or member. Reimbursement is similarly simple in public health departments, through governmental budgeting processes.

Home health services are based in inexpensive facilities, and these services are not characterized by particularly expensive technology. The ratio of labor costs to total costs decreases for those hospitals that provide primarily tertiary care and use highly specialized equipment. Labor costs relative to total costs are low in the production of drugs, durable medical equipment, eyeglasses, and other medical and surgical supplies.

In some organizations such as nursing homes, and even in certain hospitals and large multi-unit hospital systems, managers control much of the policymaking, if not the production, process.

Adaptive Capability

Organizations vary in their sensitivity to environmental conditions and in the extent to which external forces influence internal operations. In the face of rapidly changing medical technology and swings in governmental policy, many health services organizations have lacked effective adaptive mechanisms, in part because of their community service nature and loosely coupled medical work force. According to Charles Brecher and Diana Roswick, 29 hospitals in New York City, comprising 3,853 beds, could not adapt and closed their doors between 1975 and 1979. On the other hand, multi-unit for-profit hospital corporations have been able to adapt effectively in other parts of the country during that period, making substantial gains in market share and increasing their annual revenues from $4.8 billion in 1975 to $12.4 billion in 1979.

Organizing for Adaptation

James March suggests six ways in which organizations adapt, in the normal course of events. Organizations follow rules in response to new situations. They attempt to make rational choices under conditions of risk. They tend to repeat behavior that has been successful in the past and to avoid behavior that has not been successful. They make changes because of conflict among individuals or groups that represent diverse interests. They follow behaviors adopted by other organizations. And they take actions as a result of turnover (as new managers and key participants have different attitudes, abilities, and jobs).

Only large health services organizations can afford distinct, specialized units or departments to perform the adaptive functions of marketing, planning, lobbying, and cooperative action with similar organizations. In smaller organizations, many of these functions are performed directly by top managers; they may be performed indirectly as well, through joint lobbying or planning efforts with other organizations or trade associations. Smaller organizations may also buy the services of consultants to perform these adaptive functions.

Organizations vary in their need to adapt. Types of organizations facing a less turbulent environment have included group practices, hospitals in nonregulated states, and nursing homes that serve primarily middle- and high-income patients. Other health services organizations have found survival a problem because of shifting or low-income service populations and lack of access to adequate money, facilities, manpower, and management.

Varying Investment in Adaptive Capability

In the late 1970s, community hospitals became more actively involved in corporate planning; some of the larger hospitals became interested in marketing their services. The emphasis on planning was sparked by federal health planning legislation, which necessitated the formation of three-year hospital plans and required the obtaining of certificates of need from state agencies before hospitals could be reimbursed for operating expenses related to capital expenditures.

Organizations vary in the extent to which their managers provide the support services necessary to develop and adopt operational and comprehensible long-range plans. These plans commonly include information about the organization's mission, the nature of the services provided, the nature of the population being served and potential populations, and the organization's competitive situation. Plans may include timetables for future initiation, expansion, dilution, or discontinuance of services and programs, as well as details on how these changes may be accomplished. Plans may also specify the rationale for any changes, including the specification of assumptions that affect future decisions and an indication of the constraints and opportunities involved in the implementation of decisions; the plans may indicate how the constraints could be overcome or the opportunities taken advantage of.

An effective planning process must involve clinicians, as their support is usually necessary for implementation. Some organizations do not encourage participation in planning by all key groups who see themselves as affected by the plan. Without such participation, considerable planning effort may be wasted: the result is often a lengthy document, full of appendixes, which, although suitable for submission to state authorities, may be of little use in making and implementing policy decisions. Policy decisions can involve a substantial investment of funds and a possible reallocation of financial and other resources available or potentially available to the organization. Guidance in making such critical decisions is usually the reason a plan was originally created.

Varying Need for Adaptation

Organizations vary in the extent to which they are committed to adapting or organizing to adapt. Some organizations expend effort and resources in defining themselves as innovators in order to attract outside funding. Others do not. Some organizations find it easier to adapt than others, either because adaptation is an accepted policy priority or because there is confidence in the judgment of top managers and in the process by which potential adaptive behavior is evaluated.

Organizations vary in their perceptions of whether problems and opportunities exist for which adaptation is an appropriate organizational response. In some organizations, top management constantly involves key submanagers and medical officials in testing and responding to environmental pressures and groups. In others, managers and medical officials are otherwise occupied.

Organizations vary in the extent to which they take advantage of emerging trends or attempt to resist them. Faced with high allocated costs under third-party reimbursement for ambulatory services, some hospitals may choose to close or reduce these programs; others may choose to uncouple ambulatory services from inpatient services and reorganize under a separate corporate structure.

Organizations vary in the extent to which they systematically analyze the services they provide and the public's willingness to buy or to be satisfied with such services. Hospitals, group practices, and nursing homes have not been concerned with marketing in the past. As financial ceilings begin to be imposed by government and competition increases among providers, many large hospitals are beginning to examine more closely patient preferences, investigating why patients use or do not use specific services and what they like or do not like about services they do use. One indication of the current popularity of marketing in health services was the publication in 1980 of an annotated bibliography by Larry Robinson and Philip Cooper.

The bibliography includes 166 citations, with titles such as "Marketing Your Hospital," "Marketing and Enrollment Strategies for Prepaid Group Practice Plans," and "The Place of Consumer Research in Guiding Preventive Health Policies."

Organizations vary in their response to regulators. In some organizations like New York's University Hospital (see Urmy interview, Chapter 10), managers' time is freed to analyze regulations and to deal with regulators. In others, managers spend the great majority of their time responding to daily operational crises. One adaptive response to external pressure is lobbying. As Paul Feldstein points out, "some organizations seek to achieve through legislation what they cannot achieve in a competitive market—a monopoly position with regard to sale of their services and increased revenues."

Organizations vary in the extent to which they seek cooperative relationships with other organizations that provide similar services. There has been a rapid movement recently toward the creation of multi-unit systems that are integrated either horizontally or vertically. Some of the resources that are commonly shared by hospitals within such systems are data processing, exclusive domain in different clinical facilities for the same patient population, biomedical engineering, lobbying, and functional specialists in capital financing, law, and management information systems.

The 1960s and 1970s saw the development of new health services organizations that threatened the interests of existing ones. HMOs, which had existed before as prepaid group practices, have been assisted, at least some of them, by special federal legislation facilitating employee choice of plan and by grant funding. Other new types of organizations include freestanding ambulatory surgicenters, renal dialysis units, day hospitals, selfcare units, freestanding emergency units, neighborhood health centers, and community mental health centers.

Existing organizations that have been expanding rapidly include forprofit hospital corporations, nursing homes, home care organizations, and chains of dental and optometric facilities in department stores. Whether or not the current "pro-competition" strategy to give consumers more incentives to buy lower-cost services is successful, organizations with more effective adaptive capability are more likely to survive and grow in the 1980s and 1990s, while competitors fail and diminish at increasing rates.

Most health services organizations have lacked a marketing orientation to patients and potential patients. Most of them have not had to compete in terms of services or price. This has been particularly true of hospitals, the choice of which is usually made by the patient's physician rather than by the patient. As governmental payments are increasingly capped and competition among providers becomes more keen, it is expected that health services organizations will place increasing emphasis on marketing as an adaptive mechanism.

Values Integration

The values of workers in organizations are shaped by their personal history, situation, prior training, and experience. What people believe and prefer is affected by organizational characteristics such as history, size, complexity, and auspice. Some hospitals select nurses and are selected by them in large part because the hospital is owned by or affiliated with a particular religious group. What makes values integration difficult in health services organizations is a heterogeneous work force and a fragmented authority structure.

Heterogeneous Work Force

There are often significant value differences among occupational groups who have different demographic and socioeconomic characteristics but who work in the same organization. In a large hospital, the characteristics of different groups may be as follows: governing board members are largely over 50 years old, white, and male; the nursing staff and other skilled workers, such as social workers, physical therapists, and technicians, range in age and are largely white, female, and lower middle class; and the entry level staff of housekeeping, dietary, nursing, and laundry aides are mostly young, female, from lower socioeconomic backgrounds, and members of minority groups.

All of these groups working in a large not-for-profit hospital may be united by a desire (of varying intensity) to help others and will rally together in responding to patient emergencies or even to fiscal emergencies. But such groups are likely to have different responses to issues such as pay raises for nurses, allocation of an insufficient number of parking spaces among hospital staff, new medical equipment desired for the emergency services department, and provision of nonnursing services after hours by nurses. Value differences within groups may also be substantial, for example differences between surgeons and pediatricians, intensive care unit and obstetrical nurses, banker and educator board members, and black and Hispanic dietary aides.

Weak Integrative Mechanisms

Some conflict among groups, as well as among individuals, is inherent in organizations: groups will have different interests because they have different values. Some interests, for example in ambulatory or long-term care in a hospital, should be defended because they are beneficial to organizational survival and growth; others may be detrimental to survival and growth.

Integrative mechanisms include interoccupational teams, interdepartmental meetings, and social occasions. Integration is important when groups have different values but are, or should be, dependent upon each other in the production process. Integrative mechanisms are often difficult to develop because of the cost of organizing and coordinating teams and meetings. Hospital inpatient units have to be staffed on a 168-hour-per-week basis, which makes it difficult for staff members to attend meetings. Many physicians function as independent contractors and therefore have a weak commitment to or identification with the organization and with other occupational groups.

Integrative mechanisms are required as well to align the values of health services workers with those of persons who are outside the organization but who provide input to it or persons who pay for or use health services. One such mechanism is the board of directors or trustees. The governing board of an HMO is often composed partly of HMO members and users of the services, partly of local employer representatives who administer dual-choice (of health plan) arrangements for their employees, and partly of the businessmen, bankers, and lawyers who traditionally serve on hospital boards. Because of this representation, it is expected that in HMOs the voices of those who use and pay for services are more likely to be heard at policymaking levels. Whether or not such representation is actually translated into policy has not been proven.

Many health services organizations do not require managers to place heavy emphasis on integrating values of different kinds of workers, nor do they require managers to form teams and interdepartmental groups to deal with problems associated with conflicts in values. This may be because the organizations are small or because there are fewer groups with less disparate values working in them than in large, complex hospitals. Organizations with fewer and more homogeneous groups of workers include small group practices, freestanding nursing homes, and state mental hospitals. Other organizations may not require integrative mechanisms in order to respond to users and payers because their services are in high demand relative to supply; examples include group practices in smaller cities where competition is not keen and community hospitals staffed by physicians with large clienteles of middle- and upper-class patients.

Tendencies Rather than Rules

As with goal attainment, system maintenance, and adaptive capability, performance requirements relative to value integration may not differ widely between health and nonhealth organizations. Group practices and state mental hospitals tend to have more homogeneous work forces and therefore require less integration by managers. The values of salesmen and repair mechanics in a large auto dealership may conflict and need to be integrated in much the same way as conflicting values between hospital managers and floor nurses.

To the extent that the values of different occupational groups are consistent with the goals of the health services organization, there may be less conflict over the allocation of organizational resources. To the extent that organizational goals are consistent with the values of those who supply the organization with resources and pay for or use its services, then the organization may have greater access to resources or higher sales.

Health services organizations vary in the extent to which they can shield physicians and nurses from environmental pressures. In order to retain congruency between external and internal values and demands, organizations may not be able to afford managers with controversial styles or beliefs; otherwise, community groups or groups of workers may focus in any confrontation on managerial style rather than on organizational issues.

Organizational Setting

Types of health services organizations include hospitals, nursing homes, group practices, mental health centers, health maintenance organizations, day care centers, hospices, convenience clinics, maternity centers, home care agencies, and others. These types can be roughly categorized by level of care and kind of service provided, as shown in table 2.

Table 2: Categories of Health Services Organizations

Type of Service Provided	Inpatient	Outpatient (M.D.-Focused)	Community (Non–M.D.-focused)
		Acute	
General		Group practice Health maintenance organization	Home health agency Day care center
	Hospital	Convenience clinic Neighborhood health center	

Special	Maternity hospital
	Psychiatric hospital
	Eye, ear, nose,
	   throat hospital
	Orthopedic hospital
		Ambulatory surgery
		Mental health center
			Ambulance service
			Clinical labora-
			   tory

		Chronic	
General	Hospice	Day care center	Foster home Special housing
Special	Psychiatric hospital	Drug abuse clinic	

In addition to settings in which health services are provided directly, there are a large number of health-related organizations. They supply services to, or pay for, or regulate the services of direct provider organizations. Organizations that supply such services include:

—Consulting firms, accounting firms, and management consulting firms

—Universities and research organizations

—Accrediting agencies and philanthropic organizations

—Trade organizations

Organizations that pay for health services or regulate the direct provider organizations include:

—Regulatory agencies at federal, state, and local levels

—Third-party payers

—Consumer groups and legislative offices

—Large corporations and unions that purchase health insurance

The characteristics of an organization, its problems, and its history are critical in defining managerial roles and job performance. Organizations of the same type may differ more from each other than they do from different types of organizations. For example, the authors of an Association of American Medical Colleges paper, *Toward a More Contemporary Public Understanding of the Teaching Hospital*, propose five broad areas of comparison between teaching and nonteaching hospitals: multiple objectives, external controls, the medical staff, the pursuit of innovation, and cost and financing. Each of the areas is presented both as a unifying characteristic of teaching hospitals and as a differentiating characteristic among these hospitals. Some of the differences among teaching hospitals, in fact, are considerable. With regard to external controls, some teaching hospitals are independent and some are owned by universities or government. With regard to medical staff, at one extreme there are teaching hospitals in which all members of the medical staff are also salaried faculty members; at the other, medical staffs are composed mostly of physicians practicing in the community and earning almost all their income from patient fees. Effectively managing a teaching hospital that is owned by a university and has salaried faculty may require different experience, values, and skills than managing a governmental teaching hospital whose medical staff is composed mostly of physicians practicing in the community.

Effective managerial performance is also conditioned by the culture in which an organization is embedded, by the characteristics of its leading stakeholders or participants, and by the demographics of the populations served. Is a particular hospital, nursing home, HMO, or group practice located in a city, small town, or rural area? Is it in the Northeast, the South, the Midwest, or West? What role do local churches, police, and social service agencies play in the delivery of emergency services or in referrals to health providers? Which community leaders can best inform the organization as to unmet or inadequately met needs and service opportunities? What percentage of those served or potentially served by the health services organization are black, over age 65, or women of childbearing age? What are the characteristics of patients who come to the organization for service, compared to those who use other providers? Are those physicians who admit the bulk of a hospital's inpatients over or under the age of 60, and what percentage of those physicians are board-certified? Answers to these questions may determine what health services managers need to know and how they should behave.

Among for-profit corporations and physician groups, ownership is undisputed and performance requirements are clearer than they are in not-for-profit organizations. In governmental organizations, the manager's discretion is often strictly limited. Bureaucratic rules govern managerial behavior, and changing those rules is often practically impossible. In the not-for-profit organization, managers may be allowed more discretion, but at the same time they can rely less on the authority of impersonal rules. To adapt effectively to external pressures, the manager needs to gain acceptance for organizational goals among key participants (who often disagree) and then be able to implement new priorities while at the same time maintaining sufficient trust among them.

The environment that health services organizations face varies according to historical and competitive circumstances and the way in which these are perceived by key participants. Obviously, managers are better able to deal effectively with familiar situations; however, they may fail to perceive the differences between a new situation and previous ones. Or they may attempt to use customary managerial methods that do not meet current circumstances. The manager of a suburban community hospital may respond adequately to external regulatory demands and adequately meet the needs of attending physicians in their private practices. But precisely because of this experience and how it has shaped the manager's perceptions, he or she may be ill-suited to manage a hospital of similar size and services in an urban ghetto.

It may be useful to apply the performance perspective discussed in the previous sections to specific kinds of organizations so the reader can get a more concrete understanding of the concepts. The four organizations are the for-profit nursing home (late 1950s), the neighborhood health center (late 1960s), the university group practice (early 1970s), and the small-town community hospital (late 1970s).* A summary of the characteristics of these four organizations is shown in table 3.

---

*All represent ideal types based loosely on organizations in which I have worked as a health services manager. An ideal type is a typical rather than an actual organization.

Table 3: Performance Requirements, by Organization

Organization	Goals	System Maintenance	Adaptation	Values Integration
Nursing home (late 1950s)	Profit Owner needs	Referral and reimbursement	Compliance with regulations Recruitment and retention of nurses	High internal integration
Neighborhood health center (late 1960s)	Personal service and employment to local community Innovation, to professionals	Government funding Hospital affiliation	Decreases in government funding Strivings of professionals Activism of community	Pluralistic groups with conflicting goals Low internal integration
University group practice (early 1970s)	Research Teaching	Practice income	Decreases in research Need for active recruitment of patients	High internal integration, not in tune with practice requirements
Community hospital (late 1970s)	Avoid losses Satisfy medical staff Acquire high technology	Capital funding	Competitors for new technology	Conflict between manager and medical staff

The For-Profit Nursing Home
(late 1950s)

The goals of the small (60 beds), urban for-profit nursing home are to support the owner and to make a profit by providing nursing care, primarily to welfare patients.

The nursing home must meet minimum standards of governmental licensing and paying agencies; have sufficient staff with adequate training to appropriately take care of patients; have sufficient working capital so that bills can be paid while awaiting governmental reimbursement; and have managers who are able to deal with the complaints and suggestions of patients, relatives, and staff and who are willing to market services to self-paying patients and their families.

Nursing home managers must respond effectively to changes in governmental regulatory standards and changing preferences or rules of agencies that refer patients and to whom patients must be transferred. Necessary capital expenditures must be planned over time, or the nursing home must be sold before such capital expenditures have to be incurred.

The nursing home owner is the key values integrator; he or she attempts to meet the needs of patients within the constraints of the monies paid for their care. This must be done so that staff will continue to provide care of adequate quality, relatives will not be dissatisfied with care to the point of attempting to transfer the patient or complaining to the authorities, and owners will be able to make enough money to support themselves and their families and still have some free time for nonwork activities.

The Neighborhood Health Center
(late 1960s)

The primary goal of the large (215,000 M.D. visits per year) neighborhood health center is to meet the objectives and expectations of governmental funding agencies through the provision of personal service to and employment of neighborhood residents. A secondary goal is to support the professionals striving to provide innovative services in such circumstances.

Neighborhood health center management must assure adequate governmental funding to meet licensing and regulatory standards, including building codes. Another system maintenance function is assuring continued hospital affiliation and sufficiently acceptable pay and working conditions to minimize turnover of professionals.

Neighborhood health center managers must be adaptable enough to respond to reduced increases, or to decreases, in governmental funding. In case of decreases, managers can consider marketing services to persons who will pay for them, raising prices, collecting additional monies from persons already receiving services, or scaling down operations to meet the funds available, without excessive staff turnover. Managers may also have to adapt constructively to pressures from community activists and government funders to drastically alter or end a hospital affiliation that has proven critical to recruitment and retention of innovative professional and managerial staff.

Responsibility for values integration is shared among managers and clinical, unit, and department heads. Regular meetings are held among managers with unit or departmental staff. Meetings are also held by managers with representatives of government funding agencies and the affiliated hospital in order to enhance perceptions of organizational compliance with governmental objectives. Meetings are held with community groups to generate support for continued funding, to enhance perceptions of the hospital affiliation, and to remain in compliance with government objectives.

The University Group Practice
(early 1970s)*

The goal of the small group practice (fewer than ten full-time-equivalent M.D.s) in a department of medicine is to bring in revenues to offset decreases in research grants as long as this does not detract from the primary research and teaching goals of the department.

System maintenance requirements are modest: sufficient physician and support staff man-hours are needed to practice in existing facilities.

Adaptive requirements are high, because ways must be found to increase the number of patients who use the group's services. Such activities are difficult to undertake because private practitioners in the department resent such competition and because full-time physicians who are involved in teaching and research lack a competitive and practice orientation.

Integration of values is high within the group, but it is low between the group and part-time attending physicians in the same department. There is also some dissonance between the values of group physicians and the values of desired customers and their referring physicians.

The Community Hospital
(late 1970s)

The goals of the medium-sized (200–250 beds) not-for-profit community hospital in a small city include avoiding loss, assuring that the medical staff is not discontented, and acquiring new medical technology to assure market share. These goals conflict with each other in several respects. Hospital managers have traditionally reconciled acquiring new technology and avoiding financial loss by relying upon charge- and cost-based reimbursement. In an increasingly regulatory state environment, the hospital can continue to

---

*For a fuller description of the group, see A. R. Kovner, "A New Group Practice Administrator for the Department of Medicine," in *Health Services Management, A Book of Cases*, edited by A. R. Kovner and D. Neuhauser, Ann Arbor, Mi.: AUPHA Press, 1981, pp. 21–36.

acquire new technology under monopoly conditions through a lengthy and rigorous certificate of need process. Volume can be sufficiently high not to operate at a loss and to operate efficiently in terms of low unit costs, relative to costs of similar units in other hospitals.

The community hospital must maintain costing systems that assure adequate reimbursement, particularly for inpatient services in a state that regulates all hospital prices for inpatient care. It must also maintain facilities adequate for attracting and retaining medical staff and adequate technical support staff for operating highly complex medical equipment. Hospital managers must master the state bureaucratic regulatory means sufficiently well to supply the medical staff with a competitively equipped hospital. Managers must also possess sufficient sophistication, either directly or through others, to keep the hospital financially solvent.

Hospital managers can adapt effectively by reaching mutual accommodations with managers of neighboring hospitals, their own hospital's medical staff, and with government regulators concerning appropriate medical technology to be acquired and when. Managers need to know the costs of providing services at their hospital relative to costs at comparable hospitals in order to assure adequate reimbursement. If costs are not in line, then regulators must be persuaded that there are good and sufficient reasons for the higher costs, or costs must be lowered, or the hospital must change the peer group with which its costs are being compared.

Hospital managers integrate values of trustees and physicians concerning the acquisition and financing of medical technology; values of physicians and nurses concerning proper roles in providing patient care; and values among physicians concerning different priorities for the hospital's acquisition of specific medical technologies. Hospital managers integrate values of physicians and trustees with those of hospital regulators in order to assure compliance with regulations and maximum funding flows. Managers spend considerable time in developing community support for increased funding and in legitimizing new service programs or presenting the reasons for closing an old program. Acquiring such support depends in part on how influential persons in the community perceive the appropriateness and quality of patient care and amenities currently provided by the hospital.

Some of the ways in which hospital managers accomplish such value integration are the recruitment and retention of medical officials (and managers) who can adequately perform integrative roles; setting and specifying hospital goals and sharing information about them with various public groups through reports and meetings; and development of interdepartmental and interagency committes and task forces, such as planning committees at the hospital and state hospital association levels.

We shall now move from the organizational requirements and setting which bound and define managerial performance to a view of who managers are and what they do in these organizations.

II

Health Services Managers

Someone who has credibility with the professional people is needed, and I doubt that the administrator will have that kind of credibility. This is no reflection on him. . . .

Edward Pellegrino

His manner often brash, reflecting the bravado required to build so ambitiously, to attempt the different experiments, he is deeply cautious, aware of the lurking dangers of bankruptcy, of incompetence, of hubris, painfully aware that the power to persuade carries with it the responsibility not to mislead. . . .

Dorothy Levenson

There are many ways of examining what health services managers do. In this chapter, I deal with managerial job descriptions, roles, activities, skills, and persona.

Figure 5 shows the relationships among role sets, activities, skills, and functions of the manager. These relationships may be clarified by choosing any given box in the figure: for example, the box with the asterisk in it specifies the managerial planning function, which involves the role sets of motivating others, scanning, negotiating political terrain, generating and allocating resources, recruiting staff, devising work procedures, and other activities not indicated in figure 5. Managers who plan have certain communications and analytical skills, as well as demographic characteristics, beliefs, style, and personality.

Job Description

A job or position description is a way of looking at what the manager does or, by implication, does not do. The position description of an administrator of a university hospital in a larger organization is shown in figure 6. That for an administrator of a division of cardiology, in another university hospital, is shown in figure 7.

Primary functions of the university hospital administrator (figure 6) are line responsibility for day-to-day operations, direction of the activities of other administrators, liaison with professional staff, assistance with long-range planning, responsibility for compliance and financial accountability. The administrator is authorized to hire and fire, make purchases within approved budgets, and negotiate for physicians' services.

Figure 5: Managerial Functions, Role Sets, Activities,
Skills and Persona

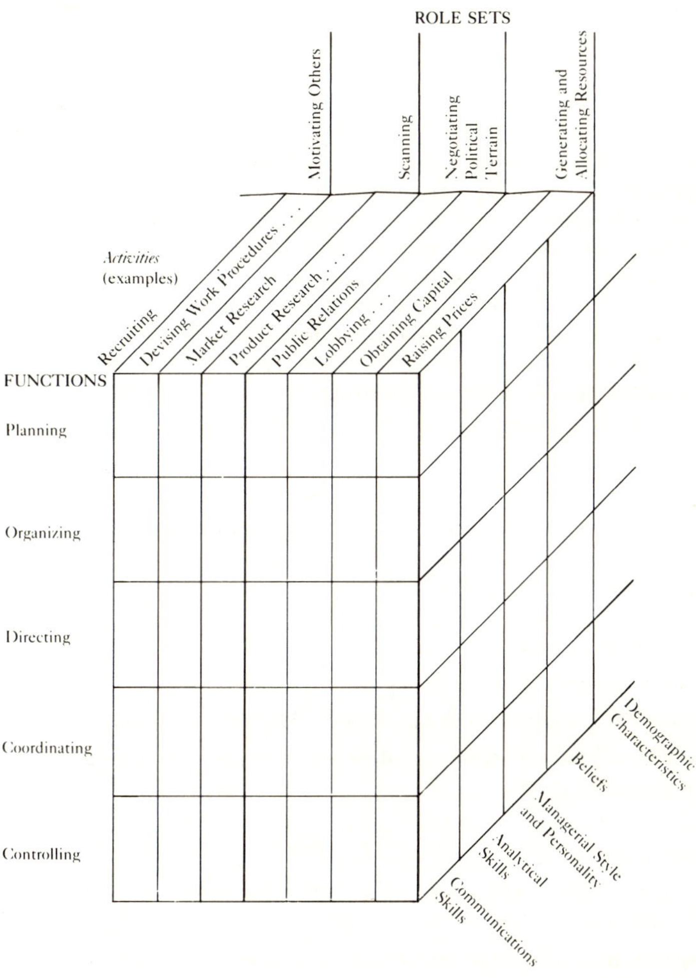

Figure 6: Position Description, Hospital Administrator, Eastern University Hospital

Position Title
Hospital Administrator

Primary Function
The administrator is responsible for all day-to-day activities of the hospital and for obtaining results in keeping with the policies and objectives established by the Executive Director of University Hospitals. The administrator directs the activities of the associate administrator, assistant administrators, medical director, and any other department, project, or function reporting directly to the administrator. The administrator maintains liaison with the professional staff and assists the Executive Director of University Hospitals and the Dean of the School of Medicine in improving and enlarging the professional staff. The administrator assists the Executive Director in developing long-range plans and programs for the hospital and is responsible for meeting required standards for licensure and hospital accreditation. The administrator has profit and loss accountability.

Authority
The administrator is authorized to employ and terminate personnel on the authorized hospital personnel budget. The administrator may purchase supplies and incur other obligations within the approved hospital operating and capital budgets and may negotiate for physicians' services for the hospital.

Accountability

—To recommend and meet budget objectives for the hospital.

—To support activities leading to operational improvements and cost reductions.

—To implement accounting controls in all sections of the hospital.

—To implement systems changes designed to improve patient care and effectiveness of hospital operations.

—To employ and maintain a stable employee work force that meets the standard of quality patient care.

—To develop coordination, cooperation, and understanding among professional staff, administration, and other hospital personnel.

—To support joint programs and cooperative activities among the University's hospitals.

—To implement programs that enhance medical staff support of the hospital.

—To regularly report to the Executive Director of University Hospital progress in meeting the goals of the hospital.

Education
A Master's Degree in Health Care Administration or Business Administration is preferred. Equivalent experience in a responsible position will be evaluated in lieu of a degree.

Continued

Figure 6: Continued

Training and Experience
A minimum of five years experience as the administrator or associate administrator of a major hospital, preferably a teaching institution, or strong experience with hospitals in a health care–related position is required.

Job Knowledge and Professional Requirements
The administrator should have complete knowledge of all aspects of modern hospital administration, with a strong professional background in organization and leadership skills. The administrator should have current knowledge of federal, state, local, and third-party and accreditation regulations which affect hospitals in the health care setting. The administrator should have the personal and leadership ability to maintain strong interpersonal relationships with professional executive personnel.

The position description for the administrator of the division of cardiology (figure 7) differs in that responsibilities and duties are listed in relation to five major functions: finance, planning, departmental organization (operations), personnel, and miscellaneous. The "miscellaneous" function includes a catchall phrase that is frequently encountered in position descriptions: "to assume all other responsibilities . . . necessary to ensure smooth operation of the Division."

Implicit in these job descriptions are managerial functions, each of which comprises a group of managerial activities. Beaufort Longest views basic managerial functions as:

—Planning, which involves the determination of objectives

—Organizing, which is the structuring of people and things to accomplish the work required to meet the objectives

—Directing, which is the stimulation of members of the organization to meet the objectives

—Coordinating, which is the conscious effort of assembling and synchronizing diverse activities and participants so that they work toward the attainment of objectives, and

—Controlling, in which the manager compares actual results with objectives to provide a measure of success or failure

The responsibilities and duties of the two managers (figures 6 and 7) can be regrouped according to Longest's functional groupings (table 4).

Figure 7: Position Description, Administrator, Division of Cardiology, Northern University Hospital

---

Title
Administrator—Division of Cardiology

Reports to
Chief and Associate Chief of Cardiology
Administrator of the Department of Medicine

RESPONSIBILITIES/DUTIES

Finances

Responsibilities:
    —The management of the Division's $1.3 million operating budget, $1.0+ million grants and funds, and $1.0+ million Medical Service Plan income.
    —The preparation of the quarterly and yearly operating budgets.
    —The preparation of the annual capital budget.
    —The preparation of research grant applications.

Duties:
    —To assemble, analyze, and distribute monthly procedure volume statistics.
    —To monitor all expenditures within the Division to ensure that expenses do not exceed budgetary guidelines.
    —To assemble and distribute reports advising of the monthly income generated from Cardiology Associates and Nuclear Cardiology.
    —To utilize the RISS computer system in budgetary and statistical analyses, in divisional demographics, and in the record-keeping function.

Planning
Responsibilities:
    —With the Chief and Associate Chief of Cardiology, short- and long-term planning to establish, analyze, and evaluate specific goals and operating standards, at the same time ensuring quality patient care.

Duties:
    —To assemble and analyze various statistics to be used as indicators in establishing and achieving goals.
    —With the Chief and Associate Chief, to set policies, procedures, and standards relating to the provision of professional services.
    —To establish policies, procedures, and standards for all other personnel/functions within the Division.
    —With the Chief and Associate Chief, to set and forecast the direction of the Division of Cardiology by selecting and implementing various management techniques.
    —To analyze and evaluate results in achieving stated short- and long-term goals and to intervene as necessary.

Departmental Organization
Responsibilities:
    —The overall efficient operation of Invasive and Non-Invasive Testing, Nuclear Cardiology, ECG, the Private-Practice Suite, and the Billing and Collection Office.

Continued

Figure 7: Continued

Duties:
—To coordinate all of the varied though interrelated activities of the Division of Cardiology and then to coordinate the Division's activities with the hospital.
—To allocate personnel and resources to areas in the Division indicating a need for temporary assistance.
—To maintain and review patient scheduling and record-keeping mechanisms, including the processing and development of medical reports.

Personnel
Responsibilities:
—The direction of supervisory, technical, and clerical staff within the Division of Cardiology.
—The staffing of all nonphysician positions within the Division.
—The final determination of yearly salary increments (based upon performance) for the nonphysician staff.

Duties:
—To recruit, terminate, transfer any member of the Division's nonphysician staff.
—With the respective administrators and supervisors, to determine and finalize all proposed year-end salary increments.

Miscellaneous
Responsibilities/Duties:
—To secure economically favorable contracts with various suppliers and vendors and to monitor the use of supplies throughout the Division.
—To initiate requests for renovations and various minor equipment enhancements.
—To initiate certificate-of-need applications as necessary.
—To prepare and distribute reports dealing with the Division of Cardiology.
—To assume all other responsibilities (not already mentioned) necessary to ensure smooth operation of the Division.

Managerial Role

Another way of conceptualizing what health services managers do is by analyzing their roles. Roles are aspects of behavior that can be abstracted for analytical purposes. Managers have to settle conflicts, lead others, and represent the organization to outside groups. These roles can be viewed as part of the manager's functional responsibilities, or they can be viewed as aspects of the managerial contribution to organizational goal attainment or system maintenance. A pictorial view of the interrelationship of roles, Longest's functions, and the organizational performance requirements specified in chapter I is shown in figure 8.

Table 4: Regrouping of Managerial Activities by Longest's Functions

Function	Hospital Administrator (see Figure 6)	Cardiology Administrator (see Figure 7)
Planning	To recommend budget objectives To support joint programs and cooperative activities among the university's hospitals	To prepare budgets and grant applications To establish specific goals and operating standards
Organizing	To support activities leading to operational improvements and cost reductions To employ and maintain a stable work force that meets the standard of quality patient care	To allocate personnel and resources to areas that need temporary assistance
Directing	To meet budget objectives To implement programs that enhance medical staff support of the hospital	To manage financial operations To manage support activities To manage personnel
Coordinating	To implement systems changes designed to improve patient care or effectiveness of hospital operations, or both To develop coordination, cooperation, and understanding among professional staff, administration, and other hospital personnel	To coordinate all of the varied, though interrelated, activities of the division and of the division with the hospital
Controlling	To implement accounting controls in all sections of the hospital To regularly report to the executive director of the hospital progress in meeting goals	To analyze and evaluate specific goals and operating standards To maintain and review patient scheduling and record-keeping mechanisms, including the processing and development of medical reports

Figure 8: Managerial Roles, Functions, and Organizational
Performance Requirements

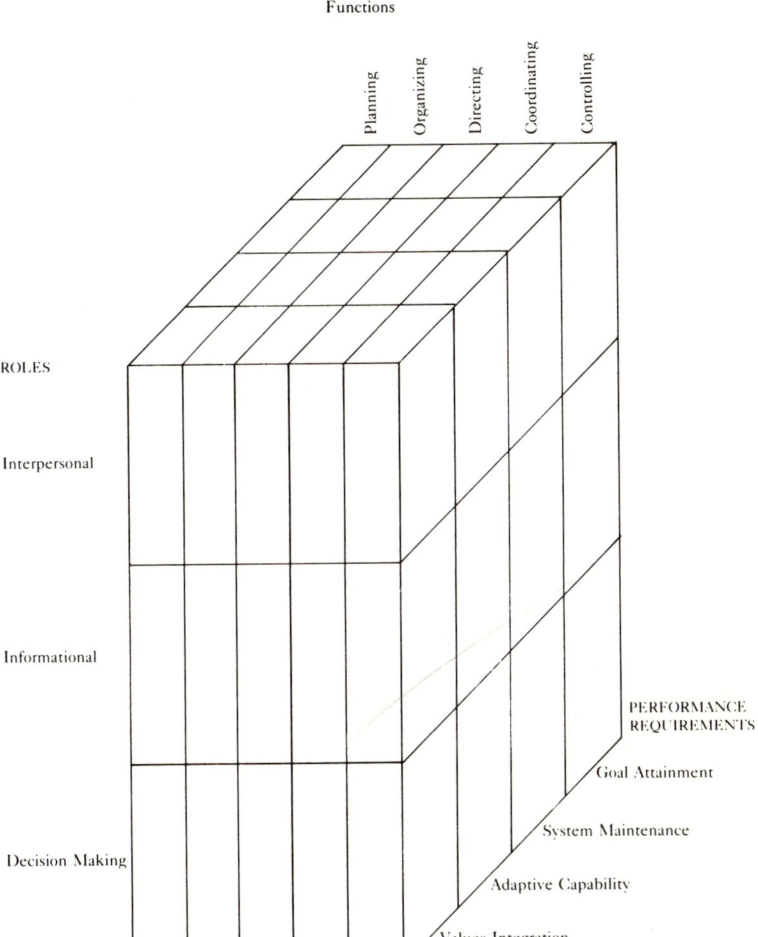

An individual's managerial roles can be abstracted from the rest of his or her behavior. This helps in understanding the managerial contribution to organizational effectiveness and the constraints upon and opportunities for managerial contributions.

Mintzberg's Managerial Roles

Henry Mintzberg has specified ten managerial roles, as shown in figure 9. He derived these roles from observing the work of five chief executives in a variety of organizations; one of them was the administrator of a large urban hospital in 1967–68. Mintzberg divides the ten roles into three role categories: interpersonal, informational, and decision-making. In other words, managers work with others, process information, and make decisions.

Of the three interpersonal roles, the first is that of *figurehead*. As figureheads, managers represent their organizations on formal occasions.

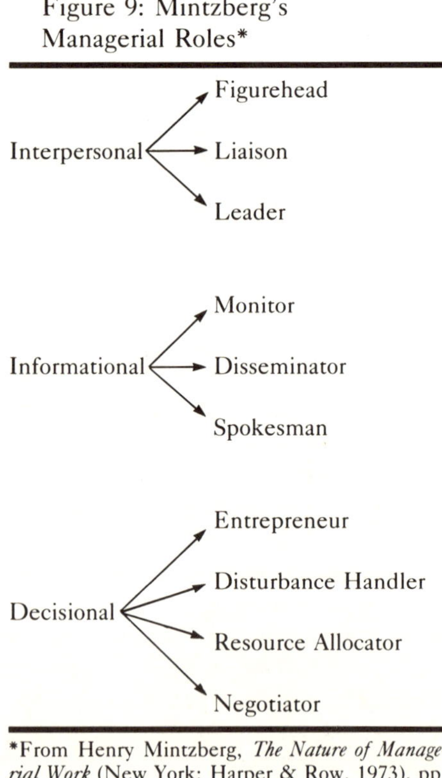

*From Henry Mintzberg, *The Nature of Managerial Work* (New York: Harper & Row, 1973), pp. 54–99.

These include opening a new facility, receiving a donation, and presenting a proposal for review by a health planning agency. A manager's photograph appears in the local newspaper as hospital representative. Managers represent their organizations at community events and before various publics, who identify the organization with the manager. Managers may be resented by co-workers for the attention paid them as figureheads by local media and persons influential in the community.

As *liaison*, the manager works with key participants in the organization and with groups and agencies upon whom the organization depends for resources. The manager establishes or inherits a communications network of people whose help can be obtained in responding to problems and opportunities. This network may include counterpart managers of similar organizations, management consultants, and regulatory, accrediting, and trade association officials. Such a peer network can assist the manager in solving local problems. For example, other managers can relate how physicians and department heads have reacted to proposed initiatives in their organizations.

The third interpersonal role is that of *leader*, which involves motivating others, setting mutual goals, and evaluating performance. The example the leader sets can serve to motivate others. Leading is a transactional, not a one-way, function. Subordinates and colleagues can give the manager information that will be valuable in his or her role of decision maker and negotiator.

Mintzberg's second set of managerial roles is informational. As *monitor*, the manager receives and collects information that enables him or her to understand the total organization more fully than participants whose responsibilities are more limited. Managers shape what information is collected, thereby affecting how physicians, nurses, and other workers perceive organizational reality.

As *disseminator*, the manager determines what information others will receive, both in writing and at meetings. Media for disseminating information include annual reports, newsletters, public relations releases, and oral presentations. The manager as *spokesman* disseminates information in person to a variety of publics. Managers speak frequently with large numbers of influential local people ranging from health planning officials to volunteers and religious leaders.

Of the four decision-making roles, the first is *entrepreneur*. Managers initiate change, develop their own ideas, or have others develop ideas for containing costs, improving services, and assuring quality. In not-for-profit and governmental health services organizations, the manager's role as entrepreneur may be limited by the perceptions and power of physicians and public officials, who may regard the manager more as a supporter of the status quo than as an initiator of change.

As *disturbance handler*, the manager takes charge when the organization is threatened. In a budget crisis, the manager often determines where cutbacks have to be made. Managers may have to respond on behalf of the organization to a strike or a work slowdown. When a powerful physician is unable to function appropriately because of alcoholism, or if a local official threatens or abuses nurses or clerks, the manager may have to step in and attempt to settle the problem fairly and decisively.

As *resource allocator*, the manager recommends and may decide where the organization will focus expenditures of effort and money. Although most health services organizations budget incrementally, policy decisions are regularly made regarding how much to spend for what type of capital equipment, which departments will be allocated what additional staff, or where reductions must be made.

The last of Mintzberg's decision-making roles is that of *negotiator*. On the organization's behalf, the manager bargains with groups and agencies regarding reimbursement, labor, and physician contracts. Negotiations are also commonly held with other local provider organizations regarding service mix decisions, joint purchasing activities, or collective bargaining.

Mintzberg argues that production managers, sales managers, and staff specialists tend to concentrate their time in different managerial roles. For the production manager (for example, the hospital department head), the decisional roles, particularly those of disturbance handler and negotiator, appear to be most important. For the sales manager (for example, the director of marketing for an HMO), the interpersonal roles of figurehead, liaison, and leader appear to be most important. For the staff specialist (such as a hospital chief financial officer), the monitor and spokesman roles appear to be most important.

There is nothing sacred about Mintzberg's ten roles. They certainly do not all apply equally well across the variety of managerial jobs and levels in various health services organizations. They can, in fact, be reconceptualized validly into eight or twelve roles. (I have condensed them into four role sets, as shown in figure 10.) The concept of managerial roles should clarify for the reader important aspects of job performance to which managers and evaluators do not pay sufficient attention. I believe that two of Mintzberg's roles warrant further discussion: those of leader and disturbance handler.

Leader

Because of the fragmented authority structure of many health services organizations, the manager, like the politician, must often lead by persuasion rather than by directive. Leadership is a relational rather than a personal characteristic, and therefore effectiveness as a leader should be measured

Figure 10: Mintzberg's Roles Reconceptualized into Role Sets

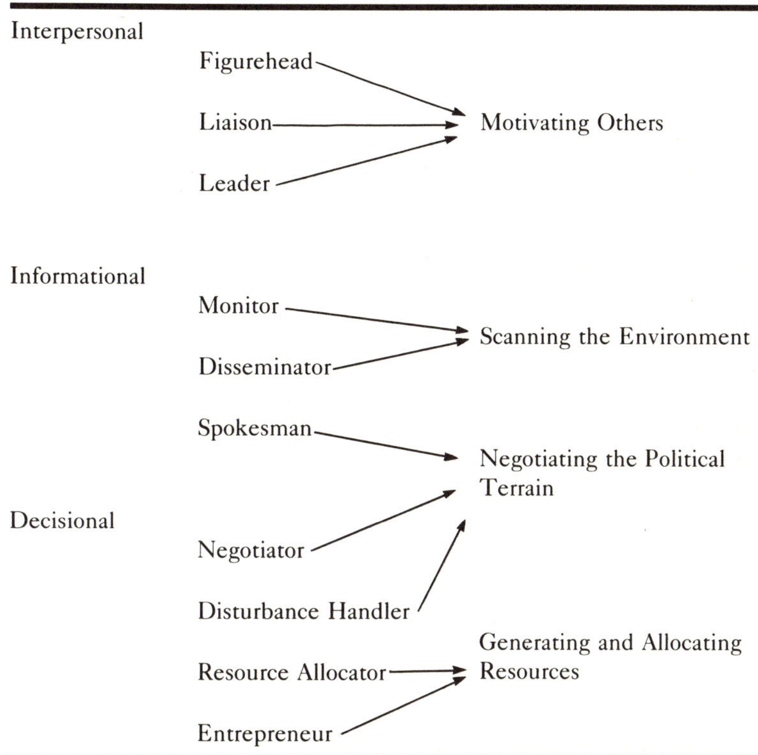

by what the followers do rather than by how the manager behaves. The health services manager, especially in governmental and not-for-profit organizations, is constantly involved in testing the positions of others inside and outside of the organization and in confronting claimants for organizational resources. The manager must constantly persuade claimants, such as physicians and nurses, that the organization has good reason for not doing what they want it to do or for doing what they object to. External regulatory agencies may compel or allow certain actions desired by claimants. What claimants want may not be equitable. Some claimants may require unequal treatment because the organization is unequally dependent upon them.

An example of such a demand is that of a hospital department head of inhalation therapy, supported by the chief of pulmonary medicine, for an increase in salary beyond the general guidelines for department heads. Either the hospital administrator must deny the request and convince these two individuals that the denial is fair, or the administrator must approve the request and convince other department heads that the increase is fair—or at least, that the decision was arrived at fairly.

Disturbance Handler

Disturbances in health services organizations sometimes involve life-and-death issues, such as providing emergency services to victims of a natural disaster, responding to a bomb threat, or confronting deranged patients or employees or aggrieved relatives. In such cases, managers must act and act appropriately as if they know what to do. Managers should plan in detail their response to possible emergency situations and should test their responses before emergencies occur.

Even when a life-or-death issue is not involved, patients and their families often have intense feelings about what they see as happening to them. For example, see Mrs. Carocalla's complaint about, and Dr. Bolles' response to, treatment of her daughter's infection (items 19 and 20, chapter 11). The mother alleges that the physician said her daughter "had to have sex to get the infected tubes." Dr. Bolles indicates that he said that "sex was only one way to get infected tubes." Clearly it is the manager's job (as disseminator, spokesman, and leader) to develop and implement rules regarding the ways patients in similar situations are dealt with and regarding how the organization will respond in the future to similar "disturbances" that are apt to occur.

Activities

Robert Allison et al. developed a list of 46 organizational activities that are performed by managers of hospitals, nursing homes, group practices, and HMOs. In their survey of six chief executives in each type of organization (24 in all), 32 of the 46 activities were determined to be crucial by one or more of the four types of executives.*

In figure 11, I have grouped these 32 activities into four role sets (see figure 10): motivating others, scanning the environment, negotiating the political terrain, and generating and allocating resources.

Motivating Others

Managers spend a great deal of their time recruiting and retaining managerial and supervisory staff and in making decisions about their rewards and

---

*It is curious to note that "advocating for patients and consumers" is not one of the 46 critical managerial activities.

Figure 11: Allison et al.: 32 Crucial Activities, Grouped by Role Set*

Motivating Others
  —Recruiting professionals and physicians
  —Decisions regarding professional and managerial salaries
  —Devising work procedures for professionals
  —Devising work procedures for nonprofessionals
  —Promoting and rewarding professionals and managers
  —Employee and management development and training
  —Disciplining professional and managerial employees
  —Motivating and directing immediate subordinates
  —Dealing with personal and interpersonal problems

Scanning the Environment
  —Market research
  —Product research
  —Long-range planning
  —Developing criteria systems to control quality
  —Decisions regarding financial and management information systems

Negotiating the Political Terrain
  —Public relations
  —Lobbying
  —Labor negotiations
  —Establishing agreements with other organizations
  —Negotiating with powerful external organizations
  —Creating and changing professional job units
  —Decisions regarding changes in decision-making and authority structure
  —Influencing decisions of Board or Owners
  —Influencing decisions made by medical staff
  —Arbitrating between internal units and departments
  —Arbitrating between policymaking groups

Generating and Allocating Resources
  —Determine buying procedures
  —Obtain long-term capital
  —Obtain working capital: collections
  —Decisions regarding maintaining building and equipment
  —Decisions regarding charges and prices for services
  —Decisions regarding new construction
  —Decisions regarding housekeeping

---

*Adapted from Robert F. Allison, William L. Dowling, and Fred C. Munson. "The Role of the Health Services Administrator and Implications for Education," in *Education for Health Administration*, vol. 2 (Ann Arbor: Health Administration Press, 1975), pp. 147–84.

promotions, work procedures, and development and training. To carry out these activities, managers use communications and analytical skills. Managers assist their subordinates in doing what is required and in doing what subordinates want to do, within organizational limits. This can be difficult if managers have not recruited their subordinates. Even when managers have recruited subordinates (and recruitment is more of an art than a science), an excellent winning percentage may be more like .600 than .850.

An example of motivating others is managerial development and training. Managers in new organizations or in new positions in existing organizations must be developed and trained by their new or existing supervisors. Such development and training can shorten the subordinate's learning process. Managers can aid those who work with them by identifying the skills that must be learned and the information that must be acquired for effective performance in the new position. Seniors can also help juniors become more aware of their own values, how they are perceived by others, and how the values of others affect their job performance.

Scanning the Environment

Effective managers scan or search the environment for potential problems and targets of opportunity. Scanning activities include market and product research, long-range planning, and quality assessment. The development of management information systems may be essential for effective scanning. In large health services organizations, scanning activities are usually performed by special units of marketing, quality assessment, development, and planning. In smaller organizations, managers may scan the environment themselves or with the assistance of subordinates or colleagues. Information about what similar organizations and managers do is available from journals, books, newsletters, and advertisements. Managers attend continuing education and trade association meetings, where colleagues and experts discuss organizational and managerial opportunities and problems. Managers visit similar organizations to learn at first hand about possible ways to improve effectiveness and efficiency. Openness to such visits is characteristic of public and not-for-profit health services organizations.

Negotiating the Political Terrain

Effective managers maintain trust and build alliances with groups and individuals. A positive political climate contributes to effective decision making and implementation. New managers must find out "who is doing what to whom" in their organization; or, put another way, "What is the ballpark in which I am playing, who are the players, and what are the rules?" Managers learn the informal organizational power structure by reading and listening. The operative rules are not always easy to ascertain—they vary by organizational setting, and they depend on the issue being discussed. Decision makers establishing a joint laundry are different from those who decide to establish a renal dialysis unit.

Activities which the manager undertakes in the area of negotiating the political terrain include public relations, lobbying, labor negotiations, influencing decisions made by governing boards and medical staffs, arbitrating between internal units and departments, and negotiating with other organizations.

Generating and Allocating Resources

Effective managers spend a great deal of time analyzing organizational efficiency and finding ways to increase revenues and decrease expenses. In doing this, managers must consider past performance in their organization, performance of like organizations, and industry standards.

Effective managers attempt to improve financial performance by making decisions about buying procedures, ways of securing long-term and working capital, building and equipment maintenance, price changes, and new construction. Effective managers attempt to understand whatever special circumstances may influence preferences among alternative standards and strategies, and they listen closely to explanations and analysis by subordinates and clinicians.

To be effective, managers continually have to make decisions about generating and using resources. This occurs as part of the budgetary process and in response to emergency or extraordinary requests. Less tangible resources, such as staff time, must also be allocated, as must resources that are less amenable to negotiation, such as space.

Skills

The manager uses communications and analytical skills in performing functions. Communications skills include reading, writing, speaking, and listening. Analytical skills include judging and deciding.

Communications Skills

Most of most managers' time is spent communicating rather than deciding. Communication skills are probably underemphasized, relative to analytic skills, in graduate programs of health services management. As Urmy indicates in his interview in Chapter 10:

> Hospital administration is not about sitting in your office with a calculator. . . .about ten percent of the job is pushing paper, bureaucratic

work. . . .Although I may have gone to six meetings and put in a ten-hour day, sometimes I feel I didn't get anything done. . . .the primary function of a hospital administrator is to provide integration and coordination within the hospital. . . .this means meetings and talking with people.

Although communicating and deciding can take place simultaneously, lengthy communication often takes place before decision making and during implementation.

Managers receive stacks of written material and have to prepare similar stacks. Some managers compensate for limited reading and writing capability by doing most of their work in person or by phone. Reading, of course, includes analyzing numbers as well as concepts or service plans. Being able to interpret numbers critically is an important skill for health service managers.

Reading and writing skills can be learned. Managers should have learned them as part of their elementary and high school educations, but unfortunately some of them have not. Many colleges and graduate schools have instituted special remedial writing courses and workshops. Speedreading courses are widely available as well.

Listening and speaking effectively are even more important for health service managers than skill in reading and writing. Many managers are not even aware that listening and speaking skills (other than public speaking) can be learned. Yet managers can learn to make focused yet personal phone calls. They can learn to conduct meetings that accomplish goals yet make attendees feel that their points of view have been listened to and their feelings have been adequately taken into account.

Listening and giving the appearance of listening are important. In a primer on consulting skills, Stanley Klion and John DeRusso attempt to teach managers how to listen better. They list the following as reasons for poor listening: lack of practice; preoccupation with one's own ideas and opinions; preoccupation with other matters; time lag (people think four times faster than they talk); and lack of common ground for understanding (people fully understand only 25 percent of what they hear).

The authors go on to list several approaches to improving listening and understanding skills. These include continually recapitulating what one is told, numbering in importance the respective points, maintaining eye contact to avoid distraction and to show interest, asking oneself how to show genuine interest, and reacting with related questions.

Analytical Skills

Perhaps more clearly identifiable than reading, writing, speaking, and listening as managerial skills are the analytical skills of judging and deciding. Ray Brown has defined judgment as knowledge ripened by experience.

Many managers feel that skill in judging and deciding can only come from experience, that it cannot be taught in school. Others argue that by analyzing and responding to managerial situations as structured cases or simulations, with students taking parts or playing roles of different participants, judgmental and decisional skills can be assessed and improved.

Before managers can judge or decide, they must, or course, be able to define a problem, gather data, structure alternatives, and calculate advantages and costs for each alternative. Each step of this problem-solving approach involves judging and deciding. For example, how valid is the manager's definition of the problem relative to key clinical chiefs' definition of it? How much time should the manager spend gathering what data?

Computational skills are also required, for example in making decisions regarding appropriate scheduling of patients for appointments, discounting the value of money over time to assess the true cost of capital financing, or pricing services to different payers so that revenues can be maximized.

Persona

The effectiveness of managers is determined as much by who they are and how they do things as by what they do. Managerial persona includes demographic characteristics, beliefs, style, and personality.

Demographic Characteristics

Managers are likely to think that how they manage rather than what population group they belong to affects how others view their contribution. However, managers tend to feel more comfortable with, and more trusting of, persons whom they see as similar to themselves.

Individuals sometimes react to managers primarily in terms of "Is the manager one of us or is he part of some group whom we dislike or fear?" The group practice administrator in a coal-mining community in Western Pennsylvania may have great difficulty gaining the trust of a union-dominated governing board of Italians and Poles when he is himself well-educated, Jewish, and from a wealthy suburb of Philadelphia.

Beliefs

People trust one another partly because of what they think others believe. "If he believes in the same things that I do, perhaps it doesn't matter so much whether I like him. I can trust him because he is likely to do what I think he should do in a particular situation for his own reasons."

Registered nurses distrust managers who they believe are interested only in "money" and who they think have little or no commitment to providing high quality patient care. They may see managers in general as holding such beliefs. Such distrust can usually be overcome only over time, as managers' beliefs become more apparent by what they say and how they behave.

Style

Managerial style is subjective, elusive, and difficult to generalize about. Some managers adopt different styles depending upon whom they are talking to. Style can be defined as the way managers perform their functions or roles and what they disclose about themselves in communication with others. Style can be learned by observing effective managers and adapting their styles to different organizational situations. The appropriateness of such adaptation depends upon the situation and the individual. Although management style may be easily differentiated and distinctly perceived by others, managers themselves may be the last to know that they are perceived as crude or overly polite, as dressing fashionably or behind the times.

Personal appearance is an aspect of style. In most organizations, physicians and nurses distrust or show little respect for a manager with a shaggy mustache, uncombed hair, no tie, and loose-fitting clothes. On the other hand, in a free clinic, such a managerial style may make performance more effective.

Formality in speech is another aspect of style. Does the manager address others initially by their first names? Does the manager initiate or encourage conversations on personal matters such as marital problems? Does the manager stand when someone enters the office? Does the manager have an open-door policy to all employees? Does the manager receive phone calls routinely during a meeting with physicians? Is the manager's desk cluttered or uncluttered? Is the manager's office formally and richly outfitted or simple and plain?

I believe that style can be learned and that it can help or hurt a manager in the performance of his or her duties. Some of my own style changes have included: more conservative dress, less talking and interrupting in meetings, and more courtesy shown to those meeting with me when I accept an important telephone call.

Managers vary in their willingness to listen at length and respond to non-work-related conversation from physicians, nurses, and employees and to listen and seek out the work and personal problems of department heads and other employees. Some managers prefer to deal with employees through the chain of command, routing personal inquiries to others unless these are from immediate subordinates. Other managers keep their doors open and welcome frequent interruptions and shifts in attention.

Some managers prefer opulent or cluttered offices; others, bare or sparsely furnished ones. Some managers place a large desk between themselves and visitors and sit in an oversized swivel chair while their visitors have low seats. Others have a work table and no desk and meet with visitors in armchairs around a low coffee table.

There is generally no right or wrong answer to a question of managerial style. Within a wide range of the acceptable, style may not significantly affect managerial job performance. Certain styles fit better in certain organizations. It is safe to asssume, however, at least in most large health services organizations, that managers should dress conservatively, show courtesy to physicians and nurses, listen, and give the appearance of listening when addressed by persons who think they have higher status. Different stakeholders in an organization expect managers to behave in different ways, and managers should attempt to understand such expectations. Many managers tune in to others' needs unconsciously and have often been selected for their jobs in part because their style fits the expectations of those who have done the selecting.

Personality

Managerial personality is an important aspect of the way managers are perceived, of whether they are trusted. Personality can have a significant impact on managerial effectiveness and survival. Of course, different people have different ideas about what is important or good.

One of my bosses had tremendous ability and intelligence, was friendly, cheerful, enthusiastic, open, and witty. Yet he had an enormous ego and was dishonest, hot-tempered, and inconsiderate. This manager read all my mail and insisted that I never close my office door. He inspired in me a determination to do only what he specifically requested—and nothing more—and to look out for myself rather than for his interest or the organization's. Yet this man was a successful manager in meeting the demands of superiors and in attracting and retaining competent staff.

Another of my bosses was able, friendly, cheerful, open, witty, honest, considerate, intelligent, and calm. If he had a big ego, he concealed it from me in our everyday relations. He obtained for me the resources necessary to accomplish my work and was always available to help with a job-related or personal problem. My response was to do anything this manager asked of me and to give much higher priority to his concerns and to the organization's. Yet this manager was perceived by some subordinates and colleagues as cold, ruthless, and insufficiently concerned with the rights of others.

It is difficult for some managers to see themselves as others see them. Sometimes only friends will be appropriately critical. Friends may be wrong about a question at issue, but they are less likely to be wrong about how others perceive the manager. Generally co-workers, especially subordinates, do not volunteer negative criticism, because they have an interest in saying what they think the manager wants to hear. Some wait for the manager to be in a relaxed mood before sharing their concerns. If the manager is always on the go, they may never see the manager in such a mood. They may feel unsure of their assessments, as assessments are often necessarily based on impressions rather than facts. Managers need to elicit from subordinates and co-workers their feelings and perceptions prior to meetings on important issues with physicians and officials upon whom managers and the organization depend.

Managers should not attempt to change themselves merely because they think some other style may be more effective or in order to please others. Often such change is not possible and, if forced, leads to worse or different results than are intended. Managers should know themselves, however, and what it is about themselves that pleases or displeases others. In this way managers can adapt better to the demands of a situation, take advantage of their natural assets, and allow for or minimize their weak points.

III

Managerial Contribution to Effective Performance in Health Services Organizations

My job is neither to control the members personally nor to run their affairs, but it is to be able to put those tigers on the stools so the act will be performed, and when a tiger is off the stool, I have to find him and get him back on the stool, or the people will want their money back.

John Danielson

Organizations are seldom formally evaluated in terms of their own specified goals. Part of the reason is the difficulty of securing agreement among the various parties of interest in an organization as to what these goals are, what acceptable standards of performance are, and who should evaluate performance and by what methods. Yet the basic problem in public organizations, according to Drucker, is not high cost, but lack of effectiveness: "Only if targets are defined can resources be allocated to this attainment, priorities and deadlines be set, and somebody be held accountable for results."

Measuring Organizational Performance

One reason for attempting to specify effective or acceptable organizational performance is to focus attention on whose organization it is. If performance is acceptable to managers, physicians, and trustees, does it matter what anyone else thinks? If it does matter, what are others going to do if they find performance unacceptable?

Another reason for developing measures of organizational performance has to do with the distribution of organizational resources. In order to adjudicate claims on resources among key groups and individuals, questions may need to be raised about the organization's purposes. For example, "What is the organization doing? How does what we do compare to what our competitors do? How does what we do compare with what our doctors, nurses, trustees, customers, and potential customers think we ought to be doing?"

Prior agreement about standards of performance facilitates agreement on performance evaluation, otherwise performance would not be measurable in terms such as "excellent, acceptable, and unacceptable." Statements such as "the hospital operated at a $100,000 surplus this year, one percent of the patients made formal complaints, and our turnover rate in nursing was down to 15 percent per year" are uncertain indicators of performance unless they can be related to agreed-upon standards and purposes. The standards of performance for which the organization and its managers are to be held accountable must be made clear in advance.

Putting Performance Requirements into Operation

Standards can be developed regarding the performance requirements of goal attainment, systems maintenance, adaptation, and values integration. Examples of these standards in operation are shown in figure 12. These standards could also be quantified in terms of desired ranges rather than points of performance.

Figure 12: Putting Performance Requirements into Operation

Goal Attainment
   —73,000 inpatient days per year (quantity of services)
   —3 percent infection rate (quality of services)
   —1,000 inpatient days per 1,000 persons in the population served (access to services)
   —Monthly meetings open to the public (process of decision making)

System Maintenance
   —Funded depreciation and a positive operating surplus (funding: capital and operating)
   —3 percent vacancy rate (staff: physicians and nurses)
   —Meet all licensing requirements (facilities)
   —Regular evaluation of managerial performance by board committee (management)

Adaptation
   —Regular and updated annual plan (environmental scanning)
   —Planning department and planning committees (specialized units with adapting mission)
   —Adequate management information system (information concerning markets, trends, market share)
   —Adequate endowment and equity capital (sufficient reserve of resources to enable adaptation)

Values Integration
   —Standards of performance set in advance for operating units (goal specification)
   —Task forces and interdepartmental committees dealing with interdepartmental problems (interdepartmental mechanisms)
   —Regular evaluation of managers based on meeting department and unit standards (accountability and control system)
   —Low absentee and turnover rates (commitment of work force to organizational performance requirements)

Certain standards, such as financial ratios, are easier to quantify than others, such as commitment of physicians and nurses to organizational performance requirements. Yet commitment *can* be quantified, in terms of turnover and absenteeism rates; unit costs per clinical service, relative to industry standards; nurses' attitudes, as measured by surveys; physician attendance at hospital social functions; and financial contributions of physicians to fund-raising campaigns. Whether the effort and cost of putting such requirements into operation and then measuring performance is "worth it" is, of course, a separate and not trivial question.

John Griffith has argued that "guidelines need to be developed for hospital performance in the face of national concern about rapidly increasing health care costs." According to him, "there should be a few, well-understood measures of hospital care—uniformly available and designed to permit each community to compare itself to other, similar communities, its state, its region, and the nation as a whole." Griffith's summary measures of hospital performance are shown in figure 13.

Figure 13: Griffith's Summary Measures of Hospital Performance*

Service Population
A. Empirically defined service populations for each of the major services of the hospital
   —Adult medical, surgical, and psychiatric services (all persons over 14 years)
   —Obstetrical services (all women 15–44 years)
   —Pediatric services (all persons 0–14 years)
   —All services population (all persons)
B. Comparable service populations for cluster hospitals—that is, those serving geographically congruent or similar areas (also expressed by services and for all services)

Quantities of Service
A. Discharge per person per year for all services, calculated as the ratio

$$\frac{\text{Annual discharges}}{\text{All services population}}$$

B. Patient days per person per year for all services, calculated as the ratio

$$\frac{\text{Annual patient days}}{\text{All services population}}$$

C. Comparable discharge and patient day rates for the cluster hospitals (detailed rates for specific services will also be available for both the hospital and its cluster)
D. Case-mix-adjusted average length of stay.

Continued

Figure 13: Continued

Cost of Services
A. Inpatient cost per person per year, calculated as the ratio

Total annual inpatient cost
All services population

B. Outpatient cost per person per year, calculated as the ratio

Total annual outpatient cost
All services population

C. Comparable inpatient and outpatient costs for the cluster hospitals

Quality
A. "Target" morbidity indicators (that is, rates of hospitalization for selected diseases, such as those known to be preventable, those believed to indicate shortages of primary care, or those reducible by public action and education)
B. "Target" mortality indicators (that is, selected specific death rates, such as infant and maternal mortality)
C. Rates of surgical procedures
    —Total inpatient surgery per person per year
    —Total outpatient surgery per person per year
    —"Target" surgical procedure rates (such as T and A rates)
D. Patient satisfaction (percent of patients satisfied) with
    —Timeliness of medical and hospital service
    —Hospital care
    —Results of hospital episode
    —Current knowledge of care resources and health needs (detailed responses, for example satisfaction with X-ray service, will also be available)
E. Comparable rates for cluster hospitals

Reasons for Not Specifying Goals

One of the difficulties in measuring organizational performance is the concept of performance objectives themselves. Charles Perrow argues that the concept of organizational goals as a major influence upon organizational behavior is "only a convenient fiction" and that much of what happens in organizations results from:

> happenstance, accidents, misunderstandings, and even random, unmotivated behavior. . . . Programs are started for a variety of vague and conflicting reasons, with the help of a lot of trivial or even accidental events. . . . Decision makers do not look for optimal solutions, have trouble discovering

what they want, and settle for the first acceptable solution that comes along, which is usually what the organization has been doing. That is, they settle so long as some important person or group doesn't want to change what the organization is doing and how the organization has been doing it.

Goal specification may not be necessary to achieving acceptable performance results in some organizations, at least not in the eyes of major contributors of resources. Specification costs may be high in relation to projected benefits, and it may be easier to accommodate diverse interests if goals are not specified. Competing members of a coalition may rarely see conflict among organizational objectives until goals are specified, at which time they may be forced to recognize and deal with the conflict. It may be easier to shift organizational direction if the proposed change does not have to meet criteria that have been previously defined and agreed to. Finally, board members, managers, and physicians may choose not to specify goals in order to avoid accountability and to maximize discretion or authority.

Results of Not Specifying Goals

Not specifying or targeting organizational performance requirements may result in lower levels of performance than would otherwise occur. By not focusing upon which goals to attain, the organization may fail to attain them. Strong members of a coalition may gain more power or resources at the expense of the weak than they would have if the goals of the weak had been considered formally by all participants. Short-run interests of a controlling coalition tend to be favored at the expense of the long-run interests of other stakeholders and potential stakeholders.

Long-term maintenance of organizational systems (that is, survival) may be threatened, or short-term organizational crises may become more frequent and more severe when performance requirements are not specified and opportunistic interests prevail.

Without such specification, it may become more difficult to make and implement policy decisions—that is, to the extent that there is disagreement regarding effective performance requirements among the controlling coalition.

Not specifying performance requirements favors retention of the present power structure. The status quo will tend to be perceived as a satisfactory level of goal attainment as long as the organization can continue to obtain necessary and appropriate inputs and sell or dispose of adequate quantities of outputs.

The environment that many health services organizations will be facing in the 1980s is expected to be more competitive and problematic. Occupational groups within these organizations may be vying more strenuously with physicians for control of organizational resources. In that case, goal specification may be perceived as less costly than direct conflict over limited resources. Evidence of a trend in this direction may be found in the startling growth of for-profit corporations, which have well-developed internal systems specifying performance requirements by unit or department.

Measuring Managerial Contribution

If there is a lack of agreement as to how or whether health services organizations should be evaluated, there must obviously be a similar lack of agreement as to how and whether the managers of these organizations should be evaluated. This is particularly true because of the difficulty of isolating the managerial contribution to organizational performance. For example, despite substantial managerial contributions, an organization may be floundering because of a hostile environment or poor decisions by previous managers. Or the reverse situation may be occurring: despite little or ineffective managerial contribution, an organization may be growing rapidly or raising quality standards and performance because of lack of competitors or excellent management in the past and excellent physicians and nurses now.

Reasons for Evaluating Managers

Reasons for evaluating health services managers are (1) to avoid setting them apart from all other employees, who are evaluated; (2) to determine continued employment and terms of employment; (3) to set prospectively agreed-upon managerial performance requirements and to assess how these requirements may be accomplished; (4) to force self-examination in regard to managerial performance and improvements that would enhance managerial performance; (5) to provide a rationale for whatever the employer wants the manager to do or for whatever the manager has done or wants to do.

A manager may be evaluated relative to what he or she has accomplished previously or relative to what managers in like organizations contribute, assuming a correlation between organizational performance and managerial performance.

Harvey's Standards for Evaluating Hospital Chief Executive Officers

James Harvey has suggested 35 standards to use in evaluating the performance of hospital chief executive officers (CEOs) (see figure 14). These standards are divided into eight categories, as follows: planning and organizing, achieving hospital objectives, quality of medical services, allocation

Figure 14: Selection from Harvey's Standards for Evaluating the
Chief Executive Officer: Planning and Organizing*

—The established planning and organizing process . . . is out in a one-year continuing cycle, which includes annual review and endorsement by the medical staff and
approval of the governing board.

—The board is not forced by external pressure to initiate or disband any program;
conversely, all new programs approved by the board are generated through the
planning process.

—Annual private poll of trustees concerning their confidence in making policy
decisions is conducted, revealing 80 percent of the board is satisfied.

—Impressions of the institution's responses to community needs, by local and state
health department officials, plus local and state health planners is generally positive. This feedback should be solicited by the chairman of the governing board.

---

*Reprinted by permission from James D. Harvey, "Evaluating the Performance of the Chief
Executive Officer," *Hospital and Health Services Administration* vol. 23 (Spring 1978): 12–13.

of services, crisis resolution, compliance with regulation, promotion of the
hospital, and self-development. Figure 14 shows the standards in the planning and organizing category.

I see several problems in applying these standards. Standards can be
met, yet performance can be poor. Validity is a problem in many evaluations, yet there may be good reason to attempt to evaluate; it is important
that the parties involved be mindful of the limitations of measurement. An
example of the limitations of Harvey's standards is that the established
planning process can be carried out within the one-year limit, can be approved by the medical staff and governing board, yet still contain inappropriate decisions and be insufficient or overdeveloped. This is less likely to
occur when the planning process is subject to such review, but Harvey's
standard does not differentiate between a planning process that is over-
lengthy, formalistic, and ineffective and one that is the opposite.

The Employer's Perspective

From an organizational point of view, evaluation is a way of communicating
to managers how superiors feel about them and of learning from managers
how they feel about superiors' assessments. This can serve as a basis for
desired changes in behavior by managers, or it may stimulate superiors to
make certain changes to enable managers to perform as desired. The evaluation process can make both superiors and managers focus on the most
important organizational objectives for the time period ahead and can
stimulate efforts to generate additional resources necessary to attain goals.

Evaluation of managers also serves as a standard for managerial evaluation of others in the organization.

Formal evaluation may not be necessary for a high level of managerial performance or for a high level of satisfaction with managerial contribution by superiors. Nor is formal evaluation of the manager a panacea for effectively adjudicating political conflict between board members and physicians. Formal evaluation can avoid misunderstandings about what constitutes satisfactory managerial performance. The process can facilitate specification of managerial performance requirements that are realistic yet responsive to organizational constraints and opportunities.

The Manager's Perspective

Just as managers have a responsibility to formally evaluate subordinates who are accountable to them for performance, they should desire a formal evaluation of their own performance. If the purpose of the evaluation is to assist managers to improve performance, then they should participate actively in the process. Evaluation should be a continuing process that is flexible enough to take into account internal and external forces constraining and facilitating performance.

The evaluation process is expensive, especially the first time. Trustees, managers, and department heads undoubtedly feel uncomfortable about an initial evaluation, whether they are being evaluated or whether they are evaluating others. The measures used may have limited validity and reliability. If the evaluation results do not square with the manager's own judgment, the cause may be faulty measurement tools or measurement bias, not necessarily the manager's faulty judgment.

Approaches to Evaluating Managers

Evaluating the Individual Manager

One approach to managerial evaluation that I helped develop as a manager begins with specifying key aspects of a top manager's job. These specifications are developed both by the manager and a board committee. Six to twelve months later, the manager and the committee separately evaluate managerial performance. [In the case of a lower-level manager, the evaluation process is developed jointly by a superior and a subordinate, in relation to written guidelines.] There should be at least three levels of performance: excellent, acceptable, and unacceptable. Further, there should be an opportunity for noting strong points or areas needing improvement in each aspect of performance.

After meeting without the manager present, the board committee summarizes its judgment and indicates to the manager the areas in which the committee agrees or disagrees with the manager's own evaluation. Then they meet together to review ways of improving managerial performance and of improving the evaluation process. The manager and the chairman of the committee sign what they have agreed to, indicating any remaining areas of disagreement and any agreement as to future plans and recommendations. The manager's evaluation is then used as an important input into superiors' decisions regarding salary and tenure. The evaluation process is confidential, as are all employee performance evaluations. Formal evaluation of a chief executive officer is done at least annually for the first few years of an appointment and again at least several months before any renewal or termination of a long-range contract.

Another version of this approach is shown in figure 15. This is the Management Supervisory Development Evaluation, which is used at the Hospital of the University of Pennsylvania. Note that the form relates results to job description and previous goal statements. Examples of present performance must be specified if ratings are other than "good." Mutually formulated goals are requested for a future period, and the evaluator is asked to identify specific efforts that will be made to assist the employee to achieve these goals. Employee comments and signature are asked for, as are requests for future assignment to other positions within the hospital or university.

Evaluating the Managerial Group

Another approach to management evaluation has recently been suggested by Dennis Pointer and Dennis Strum. This focuses on the management group rather than upon the individual manager. In a medium-sized health services organization, such a management group will normally comprise four to twelve persons. Pointer and Strum focus on the group because they assume that major events are not under the control of a single individual, and group dynamics are important when individuals' tasks are interdependent. Pointer and Strum assume that facilitating change will help the organization to be more effective.

Evaluation of the managerial group is done with the help of consultants at a one- or two-day workshop and is based on results of a 168-item survey questionnaire dealing with the processes of management. Pointer's and Strum's five processes, which are similar to Mintzberg's three role groups, are interpersonal, informational, decisional, conflict, and goal and motivational. A sample question dealing with informational processes is shown in figure 16.

There is no reason why evaluations of individual managers and of the managerial group need be mutually exclusive.

Figure 15: Hospital of the University of Pennsylvania:
Management/Supervisory Development Evaluation*

Employee's Name: ____ Position Title: _________

Department: _____________________________ Date Prepared: _______ Date of Hire: _______

Period Covered by Evaluation: From: _______   To: _______ Rating: _________________

    Assign a rating to each Development Factor and enter in the rating column of the evaluation form. After rating each factor, assign an overall rating and enter in the □ designed for that purpose.

    Up to 3 factors need not be used. The assessor may substitute other applicable factors not covered in this evaluation and assign a rating to each of these.

DEFINITIONS AND RATING PROCEDURE:

RATING	DEFINITION
O	OUTSTANDING: Performance far exceeds what is normally expected of an individual. Consistently evidences initiative, is a self-starter, and generally anticipates and plans for positive results without direction.
E	EXCELLENT: Performance exceeds what is normally expected of an individual. Generally evidences self-motivation tendencies and accomplishes tasks within scope of responsibilities.
G	GOOD: Performance meets the reasonable and usual expectations for assigned responsibilities.
S	SATISFACTORY: Performance meets minimum requirements only. Requires occasional reminding and follow-up and completes assignments under supervision.
S−	LESS THAN SATISFACTORY: Performance does not always meet minimum requirements. Requires constant and greater degree and amount of supervision and follow-up.
U	UNSATISFACTORY: Performance does not meet minimum requirements and is unacceptable. Requires constant and greater degree and amount of supervision and follow-up than can or should be expected.
X	NOT APPLICABLE TO THE POSITION: There may be certain critical dimensions of performance that are not applicable to a given position or of so little importance in operation as not to deserve a rating.
N	DO NOT KNOW ACCURATELY ENOUGH FOR RATING: It would not be expected that every manager would know enough about a subordinate's performance to rate every critical dimension of performance on the appraisal form; since no rating should be made without sufficient knowledge and information to rate, an N rating is entirely appropriate on any given item. However, it is assumed that the superior will watch in the future for evidence on these items.

*Used by permission of Hospital of the University of Pennsylvania

DEVELOPMENT FACTORS AND EVALUATION	GIVE SPECIFIC EXAMPLES OF PRESENT PERFORMANCE (Necessary if rated other than GOOD)	RATING

I. RESULTS
In relationship to job description and previous
goal statements.

II. JOB KNOWLEDGE
How has current level of technical/
professional/specialist knowledge
impacted on overall results.

III. QUANTITY OF WORK
As compared to others under your direction,
as compared to optimum level desired, as
compared against previous periods of time.

IV. QUALITY OF WORK
As compared to others under your direction,
as compared to optimum level desired, as
compared against previous periods of time.

V. FINANCIAL RESPONSIBILITY
How have dollars budgeted been managed,
have unfavorable variances been justified
by results.

VI. PERSONNEL RESPONSIBILITY
Consider examples of staff development,
delegation, discipline, grievances, turnover,
teamwork, and results generated by staff
under person's direction.

VII. DEPENDABILITY
Consider meeting of deadlines, completion
of work, attendance, punctuality, and
follow-up on areas of responsibility.

Continued

SPECIFIC GOALS FOR FUTURE PERIOD
(Mutually Formulated)

EVALUATOR STATEMENT OF COMMITMENT
(Identify specific efforts that you will engage in
to assist employee to achieve the specific goals
referenced during the coming period)

Continued

DEVELOPMENT FACTORS AND EVALUATION	GIVE SPECIFIC EXAMPLES OF PRESENT PERFORMANCE	RATING (Necessary if rated other than GOOD)
VIII. COMMUNICATIONS Consider verbal and written skills and results achieved.		
IX. LEADERSHIP AND INITIATIVE How effectively and in what situations has this person "taken charge"—what are the results.		
X. COOPERATION Consider how working relationships with supervisors, peers, and staff have impacted on results.		
XI. PLANNING How has this person prepared personally, the staff and the sphere of responsibility for future; are plans prepared?		
XII. SPECIAL FACTOR		

Continued

SPECIFIC GOALS FOR FUTURE PERIOD (Mutually Formulated)	EVALUATOR STATEMENT OF COMMITMENT (Identify specific efforts that you will engage in to assist employee to achieve the specific goals referenced during the coming period)

OVERALL RATING ☐

Continued

Indicate any interest in future assignment to other positions within the Hospital or University. If you have an interest in exploring opportunities outside of the University and would like assistance in locating a position, please indicate the type of position you have in mind.

____

____

____

____

____

____

Prepared by: _____________________ Position Title: _____________________

Reviewed by: _____________________ Position Title: _____________________

Date Discussed with Employee: _____________

Employee Comments:

Employee Signature: _________________________________ Date: _____________

*Used by permission of Hospital of the University of Pennsylvania

Figure 16: Item on Pointer's and Strum's Management Evaluation Questionnaire*

When dealing with important issues, members of the group *listen carefully* to each other. (Members ask for elaboration and clarification without being judgmental or evaluative. Members avoid interrupting one another.)

This is how it is now	(min)	1	2	3	4	5	6	7	(max)
This is how it should be		1	2	3	4	5	6	7	
How important this is in order for the group to operate effectively in performing its job		1	2	3	4	5	6	7	

---

*Reprinted by permission from Dennis D. Pointer and Dennis W. Strum, "A Framework for Management Assessment in Health Services Organizations," *Hospital and Health Services Administration* 26 (1981): 92.

IV
Educating Health Services Managers

> What is common to all true master-pupil relationships is the aware-
> ness both share that their relationship is literally priceless. . . .
> Aristotle speaks of it as a "moral type of friendship, which is not
> on fixed terms": it makes a gift or does whatever it does, as to a
> friend.
>
> *Ivan Illich*

> To what extent do the schools of health administration prepare
> beginners in the nuances, counterplays and overall strategies of ac-
> tual incidents, such as confronting clinic physicians who arrive late
> and leave early, dealing with minority militants who "liberate" the
> organization's property, and ascertaining the facts concerning a
> pharmacist charged with forging refills for Medicaid patients?
>
> *Lowell E. Bellin*
> *[paraphrased]*

How do people learn to be health services managers? Can health services management be taught? Is it a science, an art, or a craft? What can best be learned on the job? At school? Other chapters of this book deal with learning on the job. This chapter focuses on formal education.

Graduate Programs

Graduate education is increasingly being required of persons seeking employment as health services managers. This may be less true in the future, however, because large multi-unit health corporations with centralized staffing and sophisticated control systems may require less qualified persons in managerial positions of more limited scope.

There are more than 70 graduate programs in health services management in the United States. Names for such programs include health care or medical care administration, health planning and policy, hospital administration, nursing home administration, medical group practice management, and public health administration. Most graduate programs are members of the Association of University Programs in Health Administration (AUPHA). Of the AUPHA members, 19 graduate programs are housed in graduate schools of business management or public administration, 18 in schools of public health, and 24 in one or more of the following schools: business, allied health, community health, medicine, public administration, and graduate.

In the year 1981–82 students enrolled in AUPHA graduate programs numbered 5,827; 3,289 were full-time students, and 2,538 were part-time students. Of these students, 53.8 percent were women, and 13 percent were members of minority groups. In 1981, 7,297 persons applied to the programs; 3,393, or 46.5 percent, were accepted. In that year, 1,765 students were awarded masters' degrees. The 67 AUPHA programs in 1979 had 21,548 alumni, ranging from Union College's 13 to George Washington University's 1,359.

Different programs suit different persons. What decision is best for an individual depends on his or her degree of commitment to the field, age and work experience, and financial situation, as well as the availability of particular types of programs.

As of 1982, more than 53 programs had been accredited by the Accrediting Commission on Education for Health Services Administration (ACEHSA). ACEHSA is sponsored by AUPHA, together with the American College of Hospital Administrators, the American Hospital Association, and the American Public Health Association. ACEHSA requires for accreditation that the curriculum of a graduate program cover:

—Social-behavioral disciplines (economics, sociology, psychology, and political science)

—Determinants of health, disease, and desirability (the study of what health is, how it is measured, patterns and characteristics of illness, and interventions possible within a health care system)

—Elements of personal health systems and their interrelationships (evaluation, governance, financial structure, organization, function and structure, quality assessment, and social accountability)

—Management and administrative skills and their applications (organizational behavior, quantitative methods, financial management, information systems, law, strategic planning, and health regulation)

A sample curriculum is shown in table 5.

In addition to curricular requirements for accreditation, ACEHSA sets criteria in the following areas: program eligibility, resources, objectives, faculty, students and alumni, research, community service, continuing education, and program evaluation. One or more standards and a comment on each standard are developed for each area. For example, under program evaluation, ACEHSA specifies and comments upon two standards, as shown in figure 17.

Most graduate programs include an academic and a practice component, which may involve employment with or without pay in a health service organization for a period of three to twelve months. Some programs do not require a practice component at all. As the supply of program

Table 5: Sample Curriculum for the Health Administration Track:
New York University Graduate School of Public Administration

	Fall	Spring	Summer
	Full-Time Study		
One	Statistical methods for public management, planning, and policy analysis I	Microeconomics for public management planning and policy analysis	
	American public administration and its political environment	Health economics and reimbursement	
	Organization theory in a public context	Accounting and financial decision making	
	Community health and medical care	Computers in Public Management	
Two	Quantitative methods and operations management	Management and planning in health care organizations	
	Government health programs and the political process	Financial management of health organizations	
	Health care management and the law	Elective	
	Personnel management	Elective	
	Part-Time Study		
One	Statistical methods for public management, planning, and policy analysis I	Microeconomics for public management, planning and policy analysis	Organization theory in a public context
	Community health and medical care	American public administration and its political environment	
Two	Health economics and reimbursement	Accounting and financial decision making and management	
	Quantitative methods and operations management	Health care management and the law	

Continued

Table 5: Continued

	Fall	Spring	Summer
Three	Computers in public management	Government health programs and the political process	Financial management of health care organizations
	Personnel management	Management and planning in health care organizations	
Four	Elective		
	Elective		

graduates increases in relation to demand, programs may extend the formal training period to three years, one of which would be a residency.

Criteria Used to Evaluate Graduate Programs

The Student's Perspective

Applicants should select a graduate program based on school and personal criteria. School criteria may include quality and quantity of the faculty; emphasis on teaching in the program relative to other activities; commitment of the faculty to student advising; the depth, breadth, and relevance of the curriculum; the availability of field experience and placement services; and student participation in decision making. Personal criteria may include location of the school, opportunities for financial assistance and part-time work, length of the curriculum, scheduling of classes, cost, availability of student housing, and probability of admission.

The good student can probably obtain an adequate graduate education in health services management in any accredited university or school. What students learn depends on the effort they make, as well as on how others, including teachers, help. Some programs are certainly better than others for any student; and some are better than others, depending on the student.

The School's Perspective

From the school's point of view, two considerations are primary: Will the student be able to complete the program? And, Will the graduate be able to

Figure 17: Sample ACEHSA Accreditation Standard

Program Evaluation

A. There shall be a formal process for periodically evaluating the Program, involving students, faculty, alumni, practitioners, and so on, aimed at the reappraisal of program objectives and the effectiveness with which the objectives are accomplished.

   Comment: The Commission will seek evidence of a formal system for program evaluation and documentation that the system is operational, managed, and effective. There should be a process, as a component of the evaluation system, for the implementation of evaluative findings.

B. There shall be evidence that the Program considers outcome measures in relation to curricular and program objectives.

   Comment: The Commission will be seeking evidence of objective evaluation of learning outcomes; student and alumni satisfaction; long-term study of graduate performance; commentary of practitioners; and commentary of other university faculties.

---

get and keep a job in health services management? Assuming that a greater number of applicants apply than the school is willing to admit and that many applicants meet both of these criteria, priority may be given to other factors. An admissions committee may seek students who members feel will excel or lead after graduation. Little is known, however, about how to identify such future leaders. Admissions officials tend to select applicants with higher grade point averages or higher scores on special examinations (such as the Graduate Record Examination) and applicants who appear socially motivated and competent. Some programs may favor applicants who say they are committed to practice in areas that are short of personnel, such as long-term care. Sometimes a class balance is sought with regard to age, experience, ethnic background, or other demographic factors.

Applying the Criteria

How do applicants determine the likelihood that a graduate program will meet their criteria? One way is to find out whether the program is accredited and, if so, by whom. Graduate programs in health services management are located in various schools, and these schools are evaluated by different accrediting bodies. The ACEHSA will accredit graduate programs in health services management located in any school, but not all graduate programs seek such accreditation. Since many graduate programs are relatively new, and the standards for accreditation by ACEHSA are relatively difficult to meet, not all unaccredited programs are of inferior quality.

However, accreditation does certify that a given program met minimum accreditation standards at the time it was accredited.

In evaluating programs, applicants can also read appropriate brochures, talk with the program director, sit in on a few classes, and talk with faculty, preceptors, students, and alumni. Most applicants do not take sufficient advantage of these opportunities, usually because the cost of search activities is prohibitive or because they do not know whether such activities are appropriate.

Applicants can talk with program graduates and with local employers. How do employers perceive the program? Is it changing? Many graduate programs in health services management have full-time faculties of only three or four persons, thus a change of one or two faculty members might have a great impact on the graduate program.

There are partisans for locating programs in schools of business, schools of public administration, schools of public health, and so on. I believe where a program is located matters less to students than what the qualifications and experience of its faculty are. Programs in various schools may require similar courses. What tends to vary by program are the electives offered and the courses required by the school. Elective courses can often be taken in schools and departments outside the home school— sometimes even in other universities.

What many students fail to take advantage of in graduate school are learning opportunities outside the classroom. These include field projects, residencies, colloquiums with guest speakers, career seminars with alumni, volunteer work, and sharing experiences with other students who may have valuable skills and interesting work experiences and perceptions.

Undergraduate Programs

Undergraduate programs in health services administration are a relatively new development. As of 1979, 22 undergraduate programs in the United States were members of AUPHA. There were 657 graduates of these programs in that year. According to Cohen, the movement in undergraduate education began between 1965 and 1970, when a handful of programs was established to train students for entry-level positions in the health care field. Many undergraduate programs developed in a vacuum: they were isolated from one another and from the graduate programs, many of which had been established 20 years earlier.

Most of the undergraduate programs attempt to produce managers for intermediate-level positions in hospitals and for top-level positions in those health services organizations that have been found unattractive by graduates of the masters' programs. The curriculum offered by the undergraduate programs is generally similar to that offered by graduate programs. Courses that are generally required include introduction to the health care field, economics, health law, administrative theory, personnel administration, financial management, health planning, medical sociology, quantitative methods, systems analysis, and management of specific types of health care facilities.

I believe that undergraduate studies in health services management should be pursued only by students who have made up their minds early that they want a career in health services, and who intend to go into employment as soon as possible rather than into graduate study. For potential candidates for top-level management positions, education at the graduate level is clearly preferable. But for such a student to enroll in undergraduate and then graduate programs in health services management would be, I feel, a waste of educational opportunity, both because subject matter would be duplicated and because the student would lose the chance to acquire a more general education.

Continuing Education

In addition to graduate and undergraduate programs, there is a great variety of continuing education programs in health services management. They are of various lengths and cover various subjects. Some continuing education programs are offered by the graduate programs themselves. Others are offered by centers of continuing education that are freestanding or that have been sponsored by trade associations or corporations that sell equipment and services to health services organizations. Some view continuing education as helpful in improving managerial job performance because of changes in the health services field or in managers' responsibilities. Others view continuing education primarily as a fringe benefit allowing managers to take needed vacations, sometimes with their spouses.

The quality of such programs varies widely. The best recommendations as to which programs to take will come from other managers who have taken them. When such information is lacking, one should attempt to learn from trade association staff or program faculty about the particular program auspice and faculty. As an example of the size and scope of continuing education efforts, during 12 months of 1982–83, the American College of Hospital Administrators offered over 220 seminars to 7,312 attendees. The college also sponsored an annual educational conference in which 3,523 persons participated. Nonaffiliated persons comprised about 15 percent of the attendees. Examples of topics covered in 1982–83 were marketing management for health care executives, effective management of people and problems, long range planning under regulations, managing a hospital design and construction program, interpersonal skills for managers, how to expand the hospital's revenue sources, case mix management and the process, art and technique of negotiations.

A second example of continuing education is the programs conducted by Aspen Systems Corporation, a for-profit organization that specializes in health services education. According to the company's promotional literature, over 12,000 health care professionals attended over 250 seminars between 1970 and 1980. Twenty-two seminars in 12 areas were scheduled for the period of July through December 1981. The 12 areas were accounts receivable management, medical staff development, hospital systems, marketing, reorganization and development foundations, medical staff laws and bylaws, materials management, cost reimbursement, third-party coverage and payment systems, nurse recruitment, flexible budgeting, and physician compensation and contracting. All seminars were 2½ days long and cost $450 (not including air fare or hotel accommodations and meals) for a single registrant. Seminars were scheduled in desirable locations such as New Orleans; San Francisco; Key Biscayne; Las Vegas; Williamsburg; Myrtle Beach and Hilton Head, South Carolina; Rockport, Maine; Otter Rock, Oregon; and St. Thomas, Virgin Islands.

Programs of continuing education are also offered in-house by health services organizations themselves. This is particularly true of large employers such as for-profit hospital corporations. Humana, one of the largest, advertises as part of its recruitment package the benefits of its administrative management specialist program. The program is designed for young health services managers who have a master's degree in health services management or who have significant hospital experience. The program normally takes one year to complete. Each specialist is assigned by a regional personnel manager to a home hospital and is directed by a supervisor, usually the administrator of the hospital. The management program involves two kinds of activities: classroom training, which is 50 percent lecture-discussion and 50 percent workshop, and on-the-job training. In the latter, the specialist receives instruction on a specific function, observes an experienced person perform the task, performs the task himself or herself under the direction of the experienced person, and then is evaluated. Program activities include financial operations and productivity management, patient business systems, internal audit and reimbursement, and rate setting and budgeting.

Value Added

As with many elements of modern life, questions have been raised about the costs of educational programs in relation to their benefits. Would the content and cost of these programs be different if they were operated by employers instead of by freestanding centers or universities?

There has been little objective evaluation of the contributions of educational programs to managerial effectiveness, and there is little objective cost-benefit information about continuing education. Some observers argue that continuing education courses which are conducted away from where managers work are of less value than on-site learning programs, which are available to larger numbers of managers in an organization and which can be adapted to local circumstances. Many graduate programs require that students have work experience before they are admitted. Do these students do better in graduate school or stay more committed to the field?

The value of educational programs in health services management can be assessed by measuring the performance of similar managers with and without such education. Pressure for such evaluation may increase, given current demands by government to contain health services costs and given the increased competitive pressures facing programs that educate health services managers. It is doubtful, however, that consensus would be reached on the findings of such studies, because it is difficult to isolate the contribution that education makes to performance.

Part Two
The View from Below

It is the *diversity* of complex demands that makes the job a *general* management job, that makes it different, and that makes it particularly diffiicult.

John Kotter

V
Finding Your Niche

That they are in school studying management suggests concern for future jobs, but few probably planned to study business or public administration very long ago—and most have only a vague sense of the shape of their future careers.

Ross Webber

Administration in a very large hospital is an entirely different problem from management of a small institution, and the very characteristics which would make for success in the former might become a handicap in the latter.

Malcolm MacEachern

Health services managers should plan and implement their careers just as they plan and implement their activities on the job. In this chapter, I first discuss job opportunities in health services management and terms of employment; I go on to cover getting a first job, changing career direction, and improving the present situation; finally, I present other career options.

What Is Available

Health services managers are involved in general management, financial management, strategic planning, personnel and labor relations, management information systems, marketing, and statistical and policy analysis. Managers respond to demands made by community groups for service programs, gather information for compliance with governmental regulations, arbitrate and mediate among different health occupations and groups concerning the allocation of scarce resources, and assist in generating revenues from a variety of sources (for example, by organizing and implementing systems for third-party reimbursements).

Health services managers are employed by organizations that vary in size from the group practice with seven physicians to the large hospital chain of over 150 facilities. About 200,000 persons are employed as managers in the health services industry, half of them by hospitals. Other organizations that employ health services managers are nursing homes, HMOs, group practices, neighborhood health centers, and home care agencies. New types of health services organizations also employ health service managers, including freestanding ambulatory surgical centers, maternity centers, emergency centers, medical day care programs, and hospices.

For a more personal tone, "you" rather than "he or she" is used in Part Two.

Various interests sponsor or own health services organizations. These include local community groups; federal, state, and local governments; unions; business corporations; cooperatives; and physicians and other professionals. There are approximately 7,000 hospitals in the United States, 18,000 nursing homes, 8,500 group practices (over half of which employ administrators), and about 250 HMOs (organizations set up to offer various professional services in multicenters). Hospital Corporation of America, the largest for-profit hospital chain, owns over 170 hospitals in the United States and 14 in other countries, and manages approximately 150 hospitals under contract. The federal government operates over 160 Veterans' Administration, over 130 military, and about 50 Indian Health Service hospitals. Clearly there is an abundance of employment possibilites.

About 100,000 positions in hospitals are available to services managers. Patient care management positions are available in the following large departments or programs:

—Radiology and pathology

—Outpatient clinics or group practices

—Emergency services

—Nursing services

—Clinical departments (medicine, surgery, and so on)

Positions are available in the following support services:

—Finance

—Personnel and labor relations

—Public relations

—Community relations

—Grants management

—Management information services

—Marketing

—Corporate planning

Other organizations employing health services managers do not provide health services directly. These organizations regulate, pay, represent, or provide services to organizations that provide health services directly. Such organizations include over 130 Blue Cross and Blue Shield plans and a large number of private health insurance companies. Large management consulting and accounting firms with separate health divisions employ increasing numbers of health services managers. Government rate-setting and regulatory agencies have been another important employer. This includes some local health planning agencies and Professional Standards Review

Organizations that are currently being phased out but that are often reorganized under different auspices.

Numerous trade associations and voluntary organizations also employ health services managers. Blue Cross and Blue Shield of Greater New York, with $1.7 billion in income from the private sector, had 6,200 employees in 1980. The New York State Health Department's Office of Health Systems Management had a $55 million budget in 1979 and 17 bureaus in its three divisions: health care financing, standards and control, and planning and resource management.

The overall employment outlook is bright for able candidates who have the requisite skills to make an effective contribution to managing health services organizations. Not every person seeking such positions may find the job that he or she is looking for, however; many graduates do not seek careers in institutions other than hospitals or in geographic areas other than their own, where competition for jobs may be keen.

Job opportunities are expanding in the for-profit sector (such as in hospital chains and group practices), in the functional areas of not-for-profit hospitals (such as financial management and marketing), in the newer types of organizations (such as freestanding ambulatory surgical centers), in consulting firms, in trade associations, and in state regulatory agencies.

Typical positions that a recent graduate from a master's program in health services administration in the 1980s may fill include the following:

—Administrative assistant, hospital administration

—Administrative assistant, radiology

—Evening adminstrator, hospital

—Assistant administrator, nursing home

—Planning analyst, hospital planning department

—Associate director, grants and contracts, hospital financial department

—Assistant administrator, neighborhood health center

Terms of Employment

Terms of employment include pay, benefits, additional income, managerial contracts, and policies regarding conflicts of interest.

Pay

Managerial salaries in health care vary by organization, area of the country, managerial level and financial performance of the organization. According to Suzanne Seixas, who summarized the field as of September 1980 in *Money*, the starting salary for health services managers averages $15,000 in the nursing home and $20,000 elsewhere. After ten years, the health services manager will make between $25,000 and $60,000. A 1982 Meidinger Inc. survey found that median CEO/administrator salaries ranged from $60,000 in hospitals with fewer than 300 beds to $79,800 in hospitals with more than 450 beds. Manager-owners of for-profit health services organizations are unlikely to duplicate the performance of David Jones, the president of Humana Corporation, who by 1980 had personally amassed $49 million in 12 years. An AUPHA survey of 1981 graduates from master's degree programs in health services management revealed an average starting salary of $24,578.

The great majority of health services managers are paid a salary. Bonus arrangements or profit sharing are common for top executives in consulting companies and in for-profit corporations.

Benefits

Managers' benefits can be substantial in a large organization. Hospitalization and medical care benefits are usually the same for all employees, although the amount of other benefits, such as insurance, will vary with job classification and salary. Still other benefits, such as a company car or country club dues, may be available only for top managers or for the chief executive officer.

Benefits are an important aspect of managerial remuneration (they are scarcely "fringe" benefits), and in smaller organizations managers may have considerable say over what these benefits are. A most important consideration is the tax status of benefits. For example, if you receive dental benefits where you work, each dollar you would otherwise receive in salary now pays for a dollar of dental insurance premiums. If you do not have dental insurance where you work, you must pay the government 35 to 50 cents in taxes on each dollar that you receive before spending a dollar on dental services. Of course, if you have a dental plan, you can not spend those dollars on anything else; but increased dollars spent on benefits are not always deducted from salary increases, at least not after the first year of the benefit.

The list of benefits that managers can obtain is long. It includes automobile and related expenses, housing, entertainment, travel, membership dues in country clubs, even private school tuitions for children. Almost any living expense can be viewed as an expense related to a job, since you can always be working at home or while traveling. You may be talking to persons who can help the organization during all your waking hours. In that case, it might behoove the organization to pay others to do your family-related tasks such as cleaning, driving, and shopping. Some managers regard the size and furnishing of their offices and the number and pay of their assistants as benefits.

How do you obtain such benefits? Is it immoral? Do other health services managers obtain them? A hospital administrator in New Jersey in 1978 received many of the same benefits as other employees (including life insurance, the amount of which increased relative to salary) and in addition, bargained for the following benefits as conditions of accepting employment: four weeks' vacation, a car allowance, and a vested pension plan at eight percent employer's contribution. The administrator was reimbursed for travel and entertainment expenses (less than $200 per year). The hospital paid for certain journals, books, and professional memberships and allowed five days of consulting a year for other organizations, the monies from which were returned to the hospital to offset the salary.

Additional Income

The majority of health services managers can increase their salaries on a regular basis only through cost-of-living raises, which all employes get regularly if the organization is not in financial difficulty. Some organizations give managers annual merit increases or bonuses based on performance. On a one-time basis, the manager may be promoted, the job may be reclassified, or the manager may receive an "equity" raise (so called because others doing equivalent work, whether at the manager's organization or at another organization, are being paid substantially more).

If your employer wants to give you additional remuneration, it is usually possible, unless your superior is subject to organization-wide constraints. Such constraints commonly occur in the written policies of large organizations (in which case most superiors can still find a way if there is good reason, organizationally, for doing so).

If you are greatly in need of additional income and you cannot obtain more money at your present job, and yet you do not want to give the job up, you may consider working for yourself or for some other organization after hours or during vacations. (Most employers do not encourage this, however.) You may work fewer hours on the job and help out at home so that your spouse, if you have one, can earn more money.

By special arrangement with an employer, you can also teach or consult in the evenings, on weekends, or during regular working hours. Most employers would insist upon approving such activities in advance, in which case an agreement would have to be reached as to whether you may keep any funds generated from such activities or whether such funds must be returned to offset your salary.

Management Contracts

Management contracts are devices for assuring tenure in a particular position for a specified period of time. Although uncommon, they can be important for top managers (they are virtually nonexistent among beginning managers). Among the purposes of these contracts are protecting the manager and encouraging initiative.

The Massachusetts Hospital Association Task Force on Management Contracts recommended such contracts in 1979, finding that most chief executive officers are "constrained from providing innovative leadership because of the general absence of job security." A contract does not prevent the chief executive officer from being discharged quickly by the board, but "it will reduce the consequences of the sort of sudden political termination which is so prevalent in the hospital field and will provide the CEO with some security to assume greater personal risk in carrying out the goals and objectives of the hospital." A sample management contract is shown in figure 18.

Figure 18: Sample Management Contract

AGREEMENT made as of the first day of January 1978 by and between Leavis Hospital ("the Hospital"), a nonprofit corporation in such a state with such an address, and Joe B. King, chief executive officer.

WITNESSETH

WHEREAS, you were elected by the Board of Managers to the position of Executive Vice President of the Hospital in June 1976 and formally commenced your duties as such on January 1, 1977; and

WHEREAS, by action of the Board of Directors in June 1977 you were promoted to the position of President, effective July 1, 1977, and as such have acted as the Chief Executive Officer with responsibility for the overall operation and control of the affairs of the Hospital; and

WHEREAS, the Hospital desires for a period of years to be assured of the continuance of your full-time services as President.

NOW, THEREFORE, in consideration of the mutual covenants and agreements herein contained, the parties agree as follows:

1. *Term.*   The Hospital hereby employs you and you agree to serve the Hospital in the capacities and for the compensation hereafter set forth for the period beginning on the effective date of this agreement through December 21, 1981, and for such further periods as the parties may mutually agree.

2. *Duties.*   You will serve the Hospital as its President and Chief Executive Officer, with responsibility for the overall operation and control of its affairs.

3. *Compensation.*   As compensation for the services to be rendered by you hereunder, the Hospital will pay you a minimum salary of $70,000, commencing January 1, 1978, or at such higher rate as a three-member committee to be selected

Continued

Figure 18: Continued

---

from the Executive Committee may thereafter from time to time fix. Your salary shall be subject to an annual review by a three-member committee to be selected from among the Executive Committee which may determine to increase the same, but it shall not be reduced during the term of this agreement so long as you faithfully perform your duties hereunder.

4. *Other Benefits.*   In addition to the compensation provided for in paragraph 3, the Hospital will

(a) provide group term insurance on your life in an amount equal to twice the amount of your annual compensation;

(b) provide you with an automobile for use in connection with Hospital business;

(c) continue for you and your family such group health, dental, and disability coverage as is presently provided;

(d) contribute annually, or more frequently if required, to your current retirement program an amount equal to 10 percent of your current annual compensation; and

(e) reimburse you for your travel and other expenses incident to the rendering of services by you hereunder.

5. *Other Activities.*   Except as may otherwise be approved by the Board of Managers during the term of this agreement and any extension thereof, you are encouraged to participate in professional activites at the national, state, and local levels which enhance the standing of Leavis Hospital in the health community. Participation in professional activities is consistent with the terms of your appointment letter.

6. This agreement shall accrue to the benefit of and be binding upon the Hospital, its successors and assignee, and you, your heirs, and personal representatives, but your rights hereunder are personal to you and shall not be subject to voluntary or involuntary alienation, assignment, or transfer.

7. This agreement shall be governed by and construed in accordance with the laws of the state.

IN WITNESS THEREOF, the parties have executed this agreement under seal effective as of the day and year first above set forth.

LEAVIS HOSPITAL

By _______________________________

_______________________________(SEAL)

Attest: _______________________________

Management contracts are virtually unenforceable from the employer's side, in that the board cannot force a manager to manage. The contract has certain benefits for both employer and manager and raises the costs of summarily firing a manager. Whether managers can obtain such a contract depends on their bargaining power and on the preferences of the governing board for hiring a risk-taking chief executive.

Conflicts of Interest

Another aspect of managerial employment concerns participation in outside activities that employers may perceive as conflicting with work responsibilites. Managers can argue that teaching a course or consulting for another health services organization makes one a better manager and contributes to organizational effectiveness or prestige. Employers may not agree. Even if they do agree, they may still not want managers to engage in such activities, for a variety of reasons.

Conflict of interest is more commonly related to managerial decisions being affected by special interests in return for gifts or favors. This can involve decisions concerning the incomes and expenses of those who work in the organization, sell to the organization, or use the organization's services. For example, someone may want to take you out to lunch or invite you to dinner in order to get a contract or a raise. This can be acceptable if you go to a local restaurant, but not if you go to Hawaii. There are other examples: someone may wish to buy you a present, give you sports tickets, or give your spouse a job. You may wish to steer certain organizational purchases, such as insurance, to friends or relatives. Board members may wish to steer such business to their friends and relatives.

You can rationalize acting in conflict with the organization's interest by choosing not to see the conflict, arguing that "everyone else does it" or that you will not get caught, or pretending that it does not make any difference. It *does* make a difference, in terms of how you are perceived, how you perform, what you can expect from those who are accountable to you, and how you feel about yourself and your own organizational contribution. I can think of no case in which the gain is worth the cost.

The American Hospital Association's (AHA) guideline on Resolution of Conflicts of Interest recommends that a policy be adopted by hospital governing boards that any duality of interest or possible conflict of interest should be forbidden. It is suggested that managers and others should regularly fill out a questionnaire indicating any transaction, affiliations, or interests that you or members of your immediate family have taken part in or have that, when considered in conjunction with your position with or relative to your organization, might possibly constitute a conflict of interest. The AHA guide to the types of activities that may cause conflicts, and that should be fully reported, is shown in figure 19.

Figure 19: Managerial Activities That Might Cause Conflicts of Interest*

Outside Interests

To hold, directly or indirectly, a position or a material financial interest in any outside concern from which the individual has reason to believe the institution secures goods or services (including the services of buying or selling stocks, bonds, or other securities) or that provides services competitive with the institution. (The governing board may wish to define the phrase "material financial interest" in terms that can be readily determined by reference to either fair market value or a percentage of the direct or indirect ownership or beneficial interest in another organization.)

To compete, directly or indirectly, with the institution in the purchase or sale of property or property rights, interests, or services.

Outside Activities

To render directive, managerial, or consultative services to any outside concern that does business with, or competes with, the services of the institution or to render other services in competition with the institution.

Gifts, Gratuities, and Entertainment

To accept gifts, excessive entertainment, or other favors from any outside concern that does, or is seeking to do, business with, or is a competitor of, the institution under circumstances from which it might be inferred that such action was intended to influence or possibly would influence the individual in the performance of his duties. This does not include the acceptance of items of nominal or minor value that are clearly tokens of respect or friendship and not related to any particular transaction or activity of the institution. (Local law or community sensitivity may prohibit the acceptance of any gifts, entertainment, or other favors.)

Inside Information

To disclose or use information relating to the institution's business for the personal profit or advantage of the individual or his immediate family.

---

*Reprinted with permission, from *Resolution of Conflicts of Interest in Health Care Institutions*, published by the American Hospital Association, copyright 1975.

Getting a First Job

Before seeking a job, the prospective manager must decide what he or she wants to do in the field and what the chances of being able to do it are. The prospective manager should also consider how best to help himself or herself attain employment goals.

The best time to start thinking this way is not immediately before graduation. Just as one should choose a physician when one is well, you should decide what it is you want to do long before you have to actually look for a job. Test out your ideas about employment with your faculty advisor, residency preceptor, program director, fellow students, and school placement office. Remember that placement is primarily your own responsibility, not someone else's.

If you know what kind of work you want to do, examine what you need to learn to do such work. You can learn what you need to know through coursework, part-time employment, and the practice component in your educational program. After you have learned, determine how to document your skills for prospective employers.

Talk with and observe managers who hold positions that interest you. What do they like and dislike about their jobs? How do they spend their time? How are their jobs changing? What do you need to know in order to do their particular jobs well? How did they decide what they wanted to do? Has it worked out for them as they expected? What are the characteristics of managers who do and do not obtain or retain the type of job you want? What are the reasons for their success or failure? In the process of finding out what you need to know in order to learn to do a job effectively, you may find a manager who will teach you or help you, or who may even hire you or recommend you to another potential employer.

How do you identify managers with such jobs, and how do you gain access to them? Canvass everyone you know who may know someone you want to see. During two years of study in a graduate program you will meet or have occasion to meet, a variety of role models—speakers, teachers, residency preceptors, alumni, and other students. Many managers whom you wish to know will be pleased to help you. You are somebody who wants to be like them, to learn from them. This is flattering to managers who like their work and who like themselves. Your time requirements should be modest. Your questions may cause even experienced managers to rethink certain problems or to say things that surprise themselves.

What Are They Looking For?

How do you determine your chances of getting the kind of work you want? If you want to be a hospital administrator, how do you find out what available kinds of jobs can lead to this position? If an entry-level position is available, what or whom do you have to know to get that job? Other than your classmates, who is your competition likely to be?

Managers want to hire persons who can help the organization and who will make them look good—that is, somebody who is going to work hard and intelligently and not irritate important others. For most managerial jobs, this means you have to be able to listen, to absorb a great deal of information, and to tell others what you mean in a way that is clear and nonthreatening. This will be easier to do if you have a clear understanding of your own strengths and weaknesses. Dealing with others may be difficult if you are not aware of yourself as others see you. Working hard is a function of wanting to succeed, of focusing upon a particular job, of being physically and mentally fit. Not irritating others is a function of liking yourself, of not having something to prove, of enjoying other people for themselves, and of respecting others' differences.

What do you say if your resume shows you have no experience? "To get experience I have to start somewhere, which is why I am applying for this job" or "I have gone to school for a number of years; in graduate school I have been exposed to these organizations and these managers and have completed these projects. I can learn what I need to know about working in your organization fairly quickly, through orientation, observation, and discussions with peers, subordinates, and superiors."

Remember, although your competition may be stiff, you are only looking for *one* job. You have been able to complete graduate work at a good school, and, if you work hard and get along with other people, someone will benefit from hiring you.

Finding Out Where The Jobs Are

Contact your friends in the field and tell them you are looking. Get in touch with your program director, faculty advisor, and school and professional organization placement offices. Read the advertisements in local newspapers, in professional journals such as *Hospitals* (the Journal of the American Hospital Association) and the *Journal of the American Public Health Association*, and in newsletters such as that published by the American College of Hospital Administrators.

Getting An Interview

To get a job interview, start by packaging your track record in a resume. This resume should be handsome but not extravagant in appearance; it must be clear, and it should indicate results and contributions rather than merely what schools you have attended and what jobs you have held. Do not make your resume too long. For an example of a good resume, see figure 20.

When you learn of an available position, you should try to establish personal contact with the person who will determine the final applicants. It helps to have established this contact before the job becomes available. This is not always as impossible as it may seem: in large organizations, entry-level managerial positions may turn over quickly; in expanding organizations, new positions are often created. Alumni of your graduate school can tell the program director, the placement director, and you when jobs will become available.

Figure 20: Sample Resume

Salvatore Inciardi

1034 64th St.
Brooklyn, N.Y. 11219
Home #: 212-680-4714
Office #: 212-650-7784/5

Employment Experience

Mount Sinai Medical Center—1 Gustave L. Levy Place, N.Y. 10029
   December 1979–July 1980
   Administrative Resident—Department of Medicine
      Directly involved in the conversion of the General Medicine Clinics to a
      Primary Care Group Practice, assembling the group's initial budget and
      start-up timetable.
      Participated as a member of the hospital's Capital Equipment Forum. Assisted
      in the implementation of a 42-bed Unit Management pilot project.

Maimonides Medical Center—4802 10th Avenue, Brooklyn, N.Y. 11219
   January 1979–November 1979
   Assistant to the Administrator—Department of Community Medicine

Bache, Halsey, Stuart, Shields, Inc.—100 Gold Street, N.Y., N.Y. 10038
   January 1978–September 1978
   Customer Service Representative

Activities And Selected Memberships
Member, Maimonides Hospital, Community Board for Ambulatory Care,
   1979–1981
Member, American Public Health Association, 1978–1980

Education
New York University, N.Y., N.Y.: Health Policy, Planning and Administration
   Program of the Graduate School of Public Administration
   Recipient of full-tuition merit scholarship
   3.60/4.00 overall grade point average
   Master of Public Administration (Hospital Administration), 1980
Brooklyn College, CUNY, Brooklyn, N.Y.
   Economic and Finance major, Health Services minor
   3.64/4.00 overall grade point average—magna cum laude
   Bachelor of Arts, 1978

References
Furnished upon request

Often it is not possible to establish personal contact with persons who screen managerial applications. If you are replying to an advertisement and there is a person listed to write to, you can call this person and ask whether he or she would encourage you to apply. If so, ask whether you can come in and discuss the position.

Reference Check

You will be asked for references, and you should assume that these references will be checked, usually by telephone. Before listing someone as a reference, ask the person if he or she is willing to give you a positive recommendation. You should be able to screen out anyone who dislikes you enough to speak poorly of you. What continues to surprise me is the high proportion (about one in five) of negative or mediocre evaluations made by references. Most negative evaluations can be avoided by checking first with potential references.

Your references' opinions are likely to be valued highly if the potential employer knows them (either personally or by reputation), if they are perceived as speaking frankly, and if they can share direct and personal information about you because they know you well.

Being Interviewed

Try to anticipate interviewers' questions and be well prepared to answer them. Rehearse answers with your spouse and friends. Remember that you are competing with other well-qualified candidates. Be prepared to show why you can handle certain aspects of the job that are not covered in your resume. Typical questions interviewers ask include: Tell me a little about yourself, or about your experience and skills. Why do you want this job? What are your strengths and weaknesses? What kind of work do you like and don't like? What kind of results have you produced in any phase of your activities? What are you looking for in a job? What do you plan to be doing in five or ten years? Some of the questions you are asked will seem fair and appropriate; others may not.

In answering questions, be direct, brief, clear, and positive. You can build weaknesses into strengths. For example, "I am a perfectionist and am never completely satisfied with my work," or "I am very interested in results, and some people don't like that." There is nothing wrong with answering "I don't know" to questions like "What would you like to be doing in five or ten years?" This should not detract from your qualifications for the job.

Be prepared with your own questions for interviewers. Ask for information about the position and the organization. Why is the position vacant? What is the organization looking for? What are some of the problems the new occupant of the position can expect to face? What are some of the opportunities a new manager can take advantage of? To protect yourself, try to find out what risks are involved in the position.

It does not hurt to show enthusiasm about working for a particular organization and a particular management team. Do not forget your appearance. Listen well. Conduct yourself like a manager, not like a student. Remember that your interviewers are people too, with their own needs and fears. Try to key on something an interviewer is looking for that matches your strengths. If you do not match up, then perhaps the job is not right for you.

The Job Search As Education

Job hunting is time-consuming and often frustrating, especially when you are seeking employment for the first time. Rarely will you find a perfect match. In fact, as you advance in your career it becomes harder to find a good fit. What you have done and where you have been limit your employability; in addition, you target more carefully what you are looking for.

At the same time, a job search can be an excellent opportunity to learn more about yourself, to find out more about how others perceive you, and to make new contacts. One prospective employer who does not choose you may recommend you to another, whose job is a better fit. As a result of the search process you may change what you are looking for in a job because of greater self-knowledge.

Changing Career Direction

Employed managers' job options are limited by who they are, what they have done up to now, what roles they can perform, what skills they possess, and how well they can communicate these to prospective employers.

General Considerations

When you are considering a change in career direction (as well as when you are looking for a first job), ask yourself continually—until you get satisfactory answers—"What do I like to do?" and "What do I have to offer?" Some of the considerations involved in the first question are whether you prefer line or staff jobs, working in patient care or in organizations that supply or buy from patient care organizations, or working in health services or health services–related organizations at all.

Line versus Staff

Some managers prefer or are skilled at dealing with people, others with numbers and data. These characteristics may be associated with preferences as to line or staff work (although some line work involves dealing with numbers and some staff work involves dealing with people).

There are other differences between line and staff work. Line managers tend to work longer hours, their responsibility is less clearly specified, and they are generally more comfortable with ambiguous and shifting power relationships. Top line managers usually make more money and are more likely to lose their jobs than are top staff managers. Both line and staff managers have to be able to communicate with those whom they supervise or are responsible to, as well as with peers in other departments and agencies. Some managers are good at both staff and line work.

Patient Care versus Health-Related Organizations

Another question you should ask yourself is, "Do I want to work for an organization that provides services directly to patients or for one that sells to, represents, buys from, or regulates such organizations?" Some of you may be equally satisfied in either type of organization.

Working in organizations that provide services directly to patients may be the reason you wanted to enter the health services field to begin with. Managers, of course, are not usually direct providers of services; rather, they provide support services to physicians, nurses, and others directly involved in patient care. Managers do help patients by making sure that persons who provide care have the equipment, staff, and supplies to provide services effectively.

Working for a health-related organization can be like working for an organization that is not in the health care field at all. Working with consumer groups in health services may be like working with consumer groups in welfare. Regulating hospitals may be like regulating utilities. Working effectively in a health-related organization may not require you to understand fully the health services field or the production process, but it does often require you to understand the constraints and opportunities that managers of health services organizations face.

Working in an organization that sells to, represents, buys from, or regulates health services organizations can be excellent experience for working in a patient care organization. For example, experience as a health care consultant in reimbursement can make you attractive to hospitals seeking this kind of special expertise.

Health Services versus Other Services

You may feel that you have good management skills and excellent experience as a health services manager, yet you believe you can obtain greater rewards outside of health services. Perhaps you prefer health services work, but you find few opportunities available locally and you decide to explore other areas of management. The experience and skills gained in health services organizations are often transferable. Managers are managers, and financial managers are financial managers. This also applies to skilled managers and functional specialists in other sectors of the economy who wish to work in health services.

What You Have To Offer

In planning a shift in career direction, consider that every position has three phases: learning the job, mastering the job, and preparing for the next job. Even if you plan to stay with your present organization until you retire, you should consider what you would do if conditions were to change. You might lose your job or not want to work in that organization any longer. Your interests might change. Suddenly, you might have to consider what you have to sell that others are willing to buy.

Many employers ask, "What are your strengths and weaknesses?" Or "What have you accomplished that would lead us to believe that you can do for us what you say you wish to do?" As indicated in the section on getting a job, those who may hire you are interested in your contribution to results that may be transferable to their organization. What has been your contribution to increased revenues? Where have you reduced costs, obtained grants, or developed and implemented new programs? Can you prove it? What do you do really well, and how do you adjust for your weaknesses?

There is no point in lying to prospective employers about what you can or cannot do, just as there is no point in their lying to you about what they expect and how they expect you to do it. But are you flustered when someone asks you a tough question? Do you lie, exaggerate, over-defend yourself? If you have stayed in one job for many years, is this because you are lazy and not sufficiently motivated? If you have moved several times from job to job, what can you say to lead a potential employer to believe that you will not move again or that your moving was not a bad thing? What can you contribute to results in this organization? How probable is this claim, based on your past experience? Will you work comfortably with other members of their management team?

If you have certain role and skill competencies, then your potential contribution may be obvious. Some of you can steer new service proposals through the Health Services Agency, develop and implement new information systems, or negotiate expertly with unions. General managers have special skills, too. Some of you can motivate others, communicate effectively with physicians, and develop colleagues and subordinates on a managerial team.

Do not sell yourself short. If you are a hard worker, intelligent, honest, and pleasant, and if you have been doing well a job that is similar to the one you will be asked to do, say so. Do not oversell yourself, for then your prospective employer will be expecting you to deliver what you have promised. A prospective employer may be wondering why, if you are such an extraordinary manager, you are considering this job.

On the other hand, if you do not have the skills that are required for the job, you can learn to upgrade the skills you have now, and you can learn to live with your weaknesses better, at less disadvantage to yourself. You can learn more on the job or take education courses offered under a variety of auspices. You can learn, for example, how to negotiate with professionals, contain hospital costs, and implement quality assurance systems. You can learn skills in conducting meetings, writing memos and behaving appropriately as a manager.

It is important to know your strengths and weaknesses. When prospective employers turn you down for a job, they may not tell you everything they think or feel as to why. How they think you react to criticism affects what others will tell you. Look for the truth in others' criticism. Be an expert on your own weaknesses, otherwise you will never be able to successfully overcome, compensate for, or adjust to them.

Timing

How do you know when it is time to move? Is there a perfect time, which, once passed, makes a future move more difficult? Can you remain happy and challenged in one organization or in a certain job? Must managers always want more, seek more responsibility or money? If you shun greater responsibility and are happy with less (as long as you have job security), do you remain an effective manager?

I believe that each of us wants different kinds of jobs at different times in our lives. What you want at the beginning of your managerial career depends upon your upbringing, education and related debts, family responsibilities, aspirations relative to your referrent group, skills, values, and experience. Yet you may find that you have more in common with other managers on entry or in mid career or before retirement, than you have with your own preferences 20 years earlier or later.

After succeeding in a first position, most managers want greater responsibility. You may want to do what you have been trained to do and to earn more and achieve higher status, like many of your peers. Typically, this involves promotions in title, if not in position. Advancing your career usually involves changing organizations and sometimes, even changing geographic areas.

You may progress in one organization, such as a hospital, from unit manager to administrative assistant and then to assistant administrator, associate administrator, and administrator; or you may move back and forth from one kind of organization to another. In my career, I have moved from nursing home administrator to assistant hospital administrator to neighborhood health center administrator to group practice administrator to health consultant for a union to hospital administrator, with stints in academia in between and after.

What happens to your career often depends upon what happens to your boss. Plan for what is likely to happen if your boss changes—and changes suddenly. Such changes occurred frequently with my former bosses. If you are finding challenge and opportunity in your present job, and if you are adequately paid (who is ever "satisfactorily" paid?), there is certainly nothing wrong with remaining where you are.

Your needs at work change over time, and different managers have different needs and aspirations. While most of us prefer positions of higher status and responsibility, not all of us wish to pay the price in seeking and holding such positions, in learning how to perform new roles, and to use new skills effectively, in changing habits, and in altering relationships.

A good time to move on, it seems to me, is after you have spent a considerable time in one job or in one organization and feel you have pretty well accomplished what you can accomplish there. You know it, everyone else knows it, and your move will be understood and accepted. Of course a good job offer may not come along just then, but it is probably better to consider moving than not to consider it. It is certainly better to consider moving when you do not have to move, rather than when you are forced to move.

Criteria for Choosing a Job

Principal considerations for job satisfaction are location, travel required, hours of work, type of work and organization, stress, kind of boss, amount and kind of risk, and salary and benefits. In considering a job move, it is often easier to rule out what you do not want than to specify what you do want. Some managers want only to work for Boston teaching hospitals; others want to be chief executive officer of any health services or other type of organization. Others, especially younger persons, will take any job that offers an opportunity for advancement or, if unemployed, any job.

Location

The advantage of being flexible about geography is that you are more likely to find a job you are looking for if you have the whole country to look at. Given an equal number of job applicants, there is likely to be a greater number of jobs available in areas of the country where health services organizations are expanding than in areas where they are declining. As you advance in your professional career, you may find jobs at the level you desire scarce where you live because there are only so many health services organizations of the type and size you desire. A disadvantage of seeking jobs in other locations is the cost of the search.

The nonmonetary costs of relocation increase greatly as your spouse and children become attached to friends, schools, jobs, and activities. It takes time and effort in any new location to learn where everything is, not to mention how you can get anything done. If the new job does not work out, you are likely to feel much more unhappy and lonely in a place far away from familiar surroundings. On the other hand, if the new job does work out, you will have mastered a new territory, will have gained knowledge of the way services are organized in another locality, will have made more contacts, and, because of having gone through the experience, will see any next move as less intimidating.

Travel

Some managerial positions require a great deal of travel. Management consultants, for example, usually spend many nights away from home and must endure connecting and postponed flights and adjusting to (or not adjusting to) time changes. Some find such travel exciting and the change of assignments challenging and useful. Managers in multi-unit corporations may have to travel frequently to other facilities, just as managers of university hospitals may have to travel to their state's capital. The exposure to different people, ideas, and situations may improve your skills and deepen your experience.

Hours

Certain jobs, such as hospital administrator, typically require consistently long hours of work. Others, such as hospital planner, may involve intermittently long hours of work. Group practice managers or management information specialists may tend to work regular and shorter hours. For those of you whose chief pleasure in life is meaningful work, positions with long working days may be desirable. For those of you who wish to spend a great deal of your time with your family, shorter work days and work weeks will be preferable.

Type of Work and Organization

Some managers prefer to work in only one type of organization, such as a hospital or HMO, or in one type of job, such as a general or financial manager. Others prefer to work only under one type of auspice—government, not-for-profit, or for-profit. Others want a mix of all these things or certain types of jobs at certain points in their careers.

Stress

People vary in their ability to perform effectively under various types of stress. You may seek out a position involving a great deal of stress because you believe that performing under stress is part of what managers do and because you are particularly effective at working under stress. All managers have to adjudicate competing claims on organizational resources, which tends to be stressful. Jobs involving a great deal of stress often pay more and offer higher prestige; typically, they also provide less job security.

Some positions are particularly stressful because of a situation the organization faces or because of the internal political environment. As a manager, your ability to respond effectively in such situations will be affected by the amount of stress you are accustomed to, the amount of stress you are currently facing, and your support systems: you may be able to cope better with a great deal of stress at certain periods of your life than at others. Consider alternating very stressful jobs with less stressful jobs. Recognize, however, that management tends to be stressful in any case.

Boss

Often the most important criterion in evaluating a job is your boss. What kind of person do you feel comfortable working for? What limits, if any, do you place on a prospective boss? (If you do highly technical or routine work, the type of boss you have may not be a significant factor in your work, so you will have few preferences about what kind of person you work for.) You may require or prefer a boss who is highly supportive, or at least fair, or someone who will give you sufficient discretion to use your creativity and judgment and who will then recognize and reward you if your performance meets or exceeds mutually agreed-upon standards.

It may be difficult to perceive, at least during the recruitment process, what it will be like working for a boss in a given health services organization. Ask others in the organization, preferably your peers, what they think. Further, the way your boss treats you may change over time, for a variety of reasons. Bosses and managers whose styles and personalities conflict may learn to work acceptably together if each respects what the other has to contribute. Some managers can adjust to different types of superiors. Some superiors can adjust to different kinds of subordinates.

Risk

Another important job criterion is risk. This includes the possibility of not obtaining the job you want, as well as the probability of retaining a new job. Once you have a job, risk can be assessed along two dimensions: organizational risk and personal risk. Organizational risks are those faced by the organization which may result in significant reductions in size or failure to survive. Personal risks are those risks, organizational and otherwise, that you face in keeping your job. Such risks include political differences, instability of your superior, lack of loyalty of your superior, and your own lack of managerial skills or experience.

Reasons for seeking a high-risk job vary: there are greater rewards if you can perform effectively; there may be lower actual risk because of what you know or can do; or you may prefer risk for its own sake. I am assuming that preferring high risk does not mean preferring failure, but if you are willing to assume high risk, you should be able to accept failure and move on.

Consider that, in changing jobs, you may be trading a comfortable present position for one with greater responsibilities and rewards but also greater risks. Compare the ability of different organizations to survive and grow. Consider the likelihood of obtaining the job you seek. What are the consequences likely to be if your current boss finds out that you have been looking for a job and you do not get the job you want? You may then be trading *known* lesser responsibilities and rewards in the present job for *some* probability that you will be better satisfied in a new position, assuming you can obtain it and taking into consideration the costs of switching.

A useful approach in considering a job move is to use decision criteria, as planners do. If the job you prefer does not rank first, you can always change the criteria; or perhaps you will learn that the job you prefer should not rank first. This is one purpose of decision criteria.

Start by evaluating your current position in terms of what you like about it, what you do not like, and what you are indifferent to. Next, specify a set of job criteria. Third, determine how several different jobs, including your present job, meet your criteria. Steps 1, 2, and 3 of this process, for a director of planning in a large not-for-profit hospital in Los Angeles, are shown in tables 6–8.

Going through these steps will not necessarily make the choice simple. It should assist you, however, in specifying all elements necessary in such a choice and in clarifying the reasons that underlie your preferences.

Table 6: Criteria for Selecting a Job: Step 1, Current Job

Criterion	Like	Dislike	Indifferent to
Location	Move back East	Los Angeles	—
Travel	Not much	—	—
Hours of work	Regular, with some exceptions	—	—
Type of work and organization	Large not-for-profit hospital	Want the challenge of being a line manager	—
Stress	—	—	Low stress, but tolerate stress well
Type of boss	—	Boss is inconsiderate, smart, cold; steals my thunder as director of planning	—
Risk	—	—	Low risk, but willing to accept higher risk
Salary and benefits	Adequate	For the amount of effort I am willing to make, I want higher salary and benefits	—

Improving Your Present Situation

"Improving your present situation" means increasing the benefits you derive from your present position, decreasing your costs in the position, or both. Some of you may be content with your position as it is: it is not necessary to continually "improve" your situation. Furthermore, benefits and costs are perceived differently by different managers. On the benefit side, Manager A wants more money and Manager B wants more responsibility. On the cost side, Manager A wants an assistant, while Manager B wants to shuck certain functional responsibilities.

Table 7: Criteria for Selecting a Job: Step 2, Job Criteria Set

Criterion	Minimum	Reasonable	Most Desired
Location	Northeast	Northeast, large city	Boston or Philadelphia
Travel	Three days a month on a regular basis	Some travel	No regular travel
Hours of work	Want Sundays free	55–65 hours per week	45 hours per week
Type of work and organization	Planning or general management Large to medium-sized health services organization	Planning or general management Medium-sized hospital	Large hospital
Stress	Job must be doable under high stress	High amount of stress	Fair amount of stress
Type of boss	Fair Cold Unpredictable Average intelligence Trustworthy	Fair Cold Predictable Average intelligence Trustworthy	Fair Supportive Predictable High intelligence Trustworthy
Risk	High-risk organization, but employer is trustworthy Seeking new job does not jeopardize this job	Usual low risk in health services organization for job of this type Can get the job	Low risk Will get the job
Salary and benefits	Equal to current	Current plus	Current plus, plus

EXAMPLE:

Lou Baines has been working as assistant administrator at Highsmith Hospital, a 1,000-bed urban teaching institution, for three years. Baines feels that he is ready for a new job, but he likes working at Highsmith. His superior, Ned Wainwright, the associate administrator, cautions Baines to wait, assuring him that he is appreciated. Baines feels, however, that Wainwright's star is waning with Cal Calderone, M.D., chief executive officer. How can Baines improve his present position at Highsmith? Will approaching Calderone injure his present relationship with Wainwright? Can approaching Calderone hurt his prospects of finding a better job in this or another organization?

Table 8: Criteria for Selecting a Job: Step 3, Choosing Among Jobs

Criterion	Current Job	Alternate Job 1	Alternate Job 2	Alternate Job 3
	Director of Planning, Large Hospital, Los Angeles	Administrator, Medium-Sized Hospital, Small City, New York State	Consultant, Health Care Consulting Co., New York City	Planning Director, Large Hospital, Newark, N.J.
Location	Not acceptable	Acceptable	Acceptable	Acceptable
Travel	Excellent	Excellent	Not acceptable	Excellent
Hours of work	Acceptable	Acceptable	Acceptable	Acceptable
Type of work and organization	Acceptable	Excellent	Acceptable	Acceptable
Stress	Excellent	Acceptable	Acceptable	Acceptable
Type of boss	Acceptable	Excellent	Excellent	Acceptable
Risk	Excellent, will not lose this job because of search Excellent, high job security	Excellent, to obtain job Acceptable for job security	Acceptable, to obtain job Acceptable for job security	Excellent, to obtain job Excellent for job security
Salary and benefits	Acceptable	Acceptable	Excellent	Acceptable

Three options open to Baines are to do nothing, to seek another job outside of Highsmith, or to discuss the situation with Calderone. A fourth alternative, which many younger managers may ignore, is for Baines to discuss with Wainwright ways of improving his present situation. If Baines wishes to pursue this fourth option, he should prepare himself carefully. If he feels that he is being fairly paid for present responsibility, he can ask Wainwright for more responsibility. If Baines feels that he is being underpaid, he can ask for more money, or for more money as well as greater responsibility. Baines should be prepared to discuss specifics. Will Wainwright or someone else agree on a transfer of responsibilities? Does Wainwright feel that Baines has been doing well enough with his current responsibilities? It may be important for Baines to gain Wainwright's approval of suggested action before discussing it with Calderone. Calderone is certain to ask Baines what Wainwright thinks and then to discuss it with Wainwright.

Changing Aspirations or Performance?

To improve your situation, you can either change what you do, in order to get a promotion in your organization or a better job in another organization, or you can change your attitude about what you do, in order to enjoy your present responsibilities more. These two approaches tend to be mutually exclusive. Those of you who seek promotion or new employment tend to seek more and new responsibilities, while those of you who seek to become more satisfied with the way things are tend to want to do what you have been doing with less effort. There are, of course, exceptions to these tendencies. As an aspiring manager, you may spend more time pursuing advancement than contributing through hard work to organizational effectiveness. You may be satisfied with your present job, yet seek more and new responsibilities because you have been successful and you want to contribute more without spending a great deal of time planning for promotion, higher remuneration, or a job somewhere else.

Asking for More or for Less

If you do not ask, you will not receive.

Your boss may not be aware of your preferences. True, he or she may not want you to ask for more money or less responsibility—and that may be why you have not asked. If you ask for more work, Boss A may raise questions about your current job performance. If you ask for less responsibility, Boss B may consider firing you. On the other hand, your boss may be delighted to learn that you are willing to do more or to do less, because it fits in with his or her plans. The boss may be afraid that additional work will make you feel overburdened relative to peer managers; or the boss may fear that you will resent being relieved of responsibilities which, for whatever reason, the boss believes another member of the team can more effectively carry out.

What you want to avoid, however, is asking for something for which the asking or the thing itself involves high risk. Do not ask for something that may not please you later; otherwise you will lose credibility. You may want more responsibility for more areas or functions because it gives you higher status and makes you feel better than you are or better than other managers. You may think you can be responsible for the additional area or function because you do not have a clear idea of what it takes to get the job done properly. You may be comparing what you could do to what an ineffective manager is now doing, without considering why the current manager has become ineffective or what is really causing the problem.

Compelling rationales (to you, at least) for asking for "more" include: you have earned "more" based on your current and past performance; it is fair that you get more, based on what others in the organization get and what others with similar jobs in other organizations get; and your getting more will enhance organizational effectiveness. But unless the original terms of your employment were decidedly unfair or your performance has changed significantly over a specified period of time, why should the boss give you more unless there is a compelling organizational reason? It is possible, although unlikely, that the boss will grant your request primarily to make you happy. A more likely situation in which your salary is raised occurs when someone leaves. Then you may take over some of that person's responsibilities, while continuing to do everything else you do now at a slightly higher salary. Is this what you really wanted?

The Boss's Perspective

The boss must consider the alternative of not granting your request. Then will you agree that your facts regarding your performance and other managers' pay do not jibe with the boss's facts? What problems will granting your request create for your boss with other members of the top management team? Will the boss have to give them more too? Other typical arguments for not giving you more are "We can't afford it;" "We need you to continue using your energy as you are now doing;" "I'll see what I can do about it next year;" and "I'm for it, but my boss won't let me give it to you." All may be valid rationales.

If you think you are being treated unfairly do not threaten your boss unless you intend to carry out your threat. If you wish to inflict damage, you accomplish this not by threatening, but by doing whatever it is you intend to do. If you threaten to leave, your boss may ask for your resignation. It is generally better to leave on good terms with your boss; it is always better if you have decided to leave but have no new job offer in hand. Your boss may give you bad references, make your present job miserable, or use his or her discretion to give you less money or benefits on leaving than you think you are entitled to. For example, your boss may have counted the vacation days you did not take differently than you have counted them for the past four years, and now you do not have anything in writing to justify the number of days you think you are entitled to.

The best way to be paid what you think you deserve is to secure advantageous terms before accepting a position. It is generally easier to improve terms before accepting a position because your bargaining position is generally superior then. Once you are employed, it costs you more in noneconomic terms to switch jobs. These costs go down, of course, once you have an alternative job offer in hand. It is also easier for your boss to pay you more initially, because he or she can explain to others on the management team that it was necessary to give you more in order to attract you to the organization.

If you think that you are working too hard and want less responsibility, it always helps if you can find someone else who wants to do whatever it is that you do not want to do. Compelling arguments for doing less include: being able to do the rest of the job better, being willing to take less pay, and its not hurting the organization if no one does the work in question. You may want to do less for reasons of health or age or because you want to focus your effort and work more effectively in specific areas.

Your boss may not want you to do less because he or she could hire someone else who would contribute more and be paid less to do what you are doing. On the other hand, less responsibility might make you more productive. If you have contributed to the organization for many years, your boss may be constrained not to get rid of you. It is certainly partly the organization's fault if a manager fails to contribute after having been employed for several years. If the situation cannot be remedied, the manager should be assisted, financially and otherwise, in finding other employment or in accepting early retirement. However, do not count on receiving such assistance.

Other Options

Most of this book focuses on managing freestanding hospitals, group practices, HMOs, and nursing homes. At some point, health services managers may consider other options related to health services. Some of the options with which I have had personal experience are teaching and consulting. A newly emerging and important option is working in a large multi-unit hospital corporation.

Teaching

Teaching is one of the hardest jobs to do well and one of the easiest jobs to do poorly. Managers who teach management generally know what they are talking about. If you decide to teach, however, you may have difficulty communicating what you know to a live audience. There are many different ways of getting your message across. These include lecturing, dialogue, and simulation. You may have difficulty adapting your style of communication to varying levels of student competence and motivation.

For some academics, it is easy to lose touch with current operational problems and approaches to dealing with them. Ways of overcoming this include consulting for health services organizations (and teachers are often such consultants) or doing applied research in problem solving (as opposed to "pure" research, which involves hypothesis testing or theory building). Other than teaching, full-time academics do research and administrative tasks, including determining curriculum, developing and implementing standards for admission, interviewing prospective applicants, advising students, and evaluating peers.

Most teaching jobs at the graduate and undergraduate levels are available only to persons with a Ph.D. This is almost certainly true for anyone who seeks tenure. The Ph.D. commonly involves completion of two years of academic study beyond the master's degree, with the emphasis on research methods, passing a doctoral examination, and completing a thesis. Many students who are admitted to doctoral programs drop out before they finish them.

A good way to test the water is to teach part-time in a professional school or in a continuing education program such as those offered by the American College of Hospital Administrators, a state hospital association, or a health services or professional organization.

Some of the disadvantages of a career as a teacher in a professional school are scarcity of tenured positions (depending upon the discipline, the university, and the geographic area); low pay; heavy workload; pressure to publish and to do certain kinds of research; working with students who may be poorly motivated, poorly educated, and hostile; and sometimes having little power to influence school policies or program curriculums.

Some of the advantages are a great deal of control over your time, regular hours, low stress (once tenure is assured), the opportunity to satisfy your intellectual curiosity and to contribute to the store of knowledge, and working with similarly minded colleagues and with students who are highly motivated, well educated, energetic, and cooperative.

Consulting

There is a certain magic to the word "consultant." It conjures up visions of expertise, travel, being one's own boss, hiring a staff and calling oneself John Doe and Associates. Compared to the manager in a health services organization, the manager in the consulting firm is in charge of his or her own production process. Of course, the consultant also has to sell services that the other manager receives a salary for performing.

Being financially successful as a consultant requires special skills and access to markets. Merely because you know the health services "business" and how to manage health services organizations does not mean that someone will pay you for your information and skills. At the same time, your experience may be worth more than your consulting fee to some organizations.

Hiring a consultant can be like a make-or-buy, own-or-lease decision from the point of view of the buyer. Health services managers who buy consulting services may temporarily have more work to do than they can do well, or they may require the special skills and knowledge that a consultant has. Consultants are also hired for political reasons—to make recommendations that a manager has already decided upon but that might endanger his or her job or that might be perceived by others as more advantageous to the manager than to the organization. Why managers choose one consultant or consulting firm over another is a separate question.

Working in a Large or a Small Firm

If you work in somebody else's large consulting firm, you will still be working for somebody else, but you will be learning about the consulting business as a business. Some of the advantages of working in a large firm include exposure to diverse kinds of work and customers, a larger number of colleagues and mentors, and greater stability of the firm. Salaries are usually good as long as the business is there.

The disadvantages of working in a large consulting firm are similar to those of working in a large health services organization, with the added one of heavy travel. Large consulting firms do not usually want to hire other than entry-level people with one to five years' experience. A consulting firm can be a wonderful place for the young manager to begin his or her career. After working as hard and as well and as long as you know how for a number of years, either you will become a partner or you will be seeking employment elsewhere. Managers must move up or move out in consulting firms, because it is cheaper for the firm to have a large ratio of inexpensive beginners to expensive partners, and it is easier to lay off entry-level managers than to get rid of partners.

Risk is the main disadvantage in working for a small firm. If you need X thousand dollars a year to live on, where is the business going to come from? How are you going to pay your living expenses if business does not materialize? There may be cash flow problems if customers are slow in paying. Some managers do not like working in a small organization because they lack power and prestige in dealing with officials of other organizations and are often not paid the substantial benefits that large firms pay their employees.

Managing Your Own Firm

If you want to start your own consulting firm,* some decisions you must make include the following: How much money do you require yearly as a minimum? What are the skills you wish to market? How can these be marketed? To whom? Do you want to start the business alone or with a partner? With how many partners? What should be the range of the firm's overhead expenses at various income levels? What should you charge for your services?

Starting Up. The best way to start as a management consultant is with business already in hand. This is important both for your income and for your credibility. Perhaps you can arrange to get start-up work from your present employer.

Small firms often have either too little or too much business. During times of too little business, consultants have to spend more time selling. During times of too much business, consultants work longer hours, hire additional staff, turn down business, increase the backlog of work to be done, raise prices, or all of the above. All of this is easier to say than to do. Selling "cold," that is, selling to someone you do not already know, can be frustrating and wearisome for persons who prefer doing the work to selling the service. To others, however, selling is exciting and challenging. You may like people and finding ways to help them help themselves.

You should know who your customers will be before deciding to become a consultant. You should have been thinking about becoming a consultant for some time before you actually leave your present job. Should you be planning your new business on your present employer's time, marketing or at least engaging in premarketing efforts for your new consulting firm? You can rationalize such behavior by arguing that you have been underpaid by your present employers for several years now. Whatever your rationalization, no present employer is likely to agree, however, unless this is part of a severance agreement that has been agreed to by both parties.

---

*Although it is rare for graduates of a master's program to begin work on their own as management consultants in health services, I know of at least four of my former students who have done so successfully.

Who your new firm's customers will be depends on your skills and contracts and upon which organizations can afford and will demand your services. General management skills can be difficult to sell. Organizations are paying their own managers to manage and will seldom call in an outsider as a general management consultant, regardless of potential organizational benefits. Management audits are often made before an organization decides whether or not to fire its present management team. In such a case, the neutrality of a consulting firm is valuable. The large, experienced consulting firm is generally preferred to the small new firm, both because the large firm is perceived to be more neutral and because the usually higher cost of the large firm's contract is small relative to the perceived benefits.

What You Have To Sell. Managers can sell an organization their skills in doing tasks and performing roles for like organizations. (You must be able to document these skills.) Selling is a skill. Listening is a skill. Writing, public speaking, and knowledge of sources of information are skills. Selling yourself to clients involves persuading them that they have needs and that you can fill them or responding to needs clients know they have and persuading them to select your firm to meet these needs. You must also find clients who can afford and who are willing to pay for the services your consulting firm provides.

What clients want is work of acceptable quality at a reasonable cost within a specified period of time. They are more likely to believe you can perform if your firm has already done similar work and if you come highly recommended by a respected client. For this reason, new consultants are unlikely to obtain large, important contracts unless they have performed similar work previously as salaried employees.

New consultants are more likely to obtain small, unimportant (to the purchaser) contracts. You are likely to bid successfully for small contracts if your price is cheaper and if you may get the job done faster and by more experienced people than a larger firm. Of course, a few small, "unimportant" contracts may be enough to support one or two consultants for some time.

Solo versus Partnership Practice. As a new consultant, you must decide early on whether you want to be in business for yourself or with a partner or partners. There is no reason to have partners if you can generate enough business on your own and if you can hire competent people to perform additional work. The advantage of being the owner of a business is that if it succeeds, you obtain most of the economic and status benefits. Some individuals who would otherwise blame their lack of success on others or worry about having the benefits of their effort going to others rise to the challenge of having the entire business depending on them.

An advantage of having partners is that they may have skills that are complementary to yours. This should give the firm access to markets that no one partner could reach on his or her own. You may work more effectively with a partner than alone. For the new consultant, having a partner may enable you to take some time off without hurting business. You can learn from partners and benefit from their criticism.

One disadvantage that often comes with partners is their spouses, who may differ from the partners about the costs that are incurred and the benefits that should accrue to each. Partners may have different preferences about the proportion of monies paid out in salaries versus earnings retained in the business or loaned to the business. They may differ concerning the luxury of their offices or the benefits paid to employees.

If the new consulting firm is successful, and most new firms are not, then the consultant has to worry about how large the firm should be. Operating a consulting firm with two partners and eight employees in one office is quite different from operating a firm with tens of partners, hundreds of employees, and offices in several states.

Some consultants work out of their homes. They meet the client in the client's office and part of their house expenses may become tax-deductible. Such expenses include part of the rent or mortgage, light, heat, and telephone. All they may require in start-up expenses is the cost of stationery and business cards. Many part-time consultants have other jobs and operate in this way.

Other consultants cannot work effectively in their own homes. Renting office space can be a problem. How much of what kind of space a consultant needs is related to how much business he or she will have, and that cannot be forecast accurately. There is a great deal of variability in a small firm's revenues, and sometimes office space must be leased for long periods of time. Prices for office space can change rapidly, and moving is costly and inconvenient.

Similar questions arise in regard to hiring full-time or part-time staff. Full-time staff are desirable because they are more available during, and sometimes after, working hours, and they can be expected to have greater commitment to the firm and to the business. Full-time emloyees cost more however, because they may have to be paid benefits, which part-time employees do not require, and there may not be enough work to occupy them fully.

What to Charge. Another decision consultants have to make early on is how much to charge for their services. Basically, charges are made up of an hourly rate for the consultants' time, plus expenses incurred in doing the work. One approach is to prorate the salary you would be making if you were employed as a manager. A $25,000 salary plus 15 percent benefits, or $28,750, is about $115 per day, assuming 250 working days. This sounds like a reasonable charge. However, this charge is based on the assumption that your consulting firm incurs no overhead (marketing and other expenses) and that it has 250 days of paid work during the year. Consultants who are in demand may be charging $115 an hour, not $115 per day. Different customers may be willing to pay different amounts for the same work. You may be willing to do certain jobs at a loss because they may lead to other, more remunerative contracts or to similar contracts that you can do at one-half the cost since they are simply an adaptation of previous work.

Market Positioning. If what you have to sell is primarily knowledge of or experience in a specific area, such as maneuvering proposals through the state regulatory process or helping to start up and operate a hospital-based group practice, then there may be an advantage to concentrating your consulting efforts in only a few technical areas. It may make sense for a small firm or an individual to focus on a problem area or client group that is too small for large firms to address or to serve profitably.

Consulting jobs in small firms may include preparing a patient booklet or annual report or improving the billings and collection systems of small to medium-sized hospitals or large group practices. Client groups may include nursing homes, group practices, rural hospitals, and small HMOs. You can create new opportunities, however, by becoming expert in dealing with new problems or with old problems that new health services organizations face. Such opportunities may result from federal legislation, such as that which created Professional Standards Review Organizations, or from the development and expansion of new services programs, such as free-standing convenience clinics or HMOs.

Managing in Multi-Unit Hospital Corporations

One of the significant new developments in health services has been the rapid and recent growth of multi-unit, and specifically of for-profit, hospital and related health services corporations. About 1,000 of the 7,000 hospitals in the United States are operated for profit. About half of these are owned by large corporations that specialize in hospital ownership or management. In addition, as of 1979, profit-making hospital corporations managed under contract about 300 not-for-profit hospitals. Most for-profit hospitals have from 100 to 250 beds, with few outpatient facilities other than an emergency room. Most are located in the south, the southeast, and on the Pacific coast. As of 1979, the four largest hospital corporations in the country were Hospital Corporation of America and Humana, each with a gross revenue of over $1 billion, and American Medical International and Hospital Affiliates International, with gross revenues of approximately $500 million each.

There are also not-for-profit and public multihospital corporations. These have not been growing as rapidly as the for-profits. Examples of not-for-profit multihospital corporations are the Sisters of Mercy Health Corporation, Samaritan Health Service, Intermountain Health Care, Inc., and the Lutheran Hospital Society of Southern California. The not-for-profit Kaiser-Permanente HMO system includes 24 hospitals that serve almost 4 million Americans. In the public sector, the federal government has about 170 Veterans Administration, 131 military, and 50 Indian hospitals.

There are also large multi-unit corporations that focus on a particular kind of care, such as nursing homes, psychiatric and alcoholic care at home, and kidney dialysis services. Large corporations also sell and manage a variety of products and services that are sold to hospitals, to other health services organizations, and to the public. These services include mobile CAT scanning, cardiopulmonary testing, industrial health screening, rehabilitation counselling, dental care, weight control clinics, comprehensive prepaid HMO programs, physician house calls, and laboratory and emergency services. Arnold Relman estimates revenues of for-profit health services and related organizations—"the new medical-industrial complex"—to be between $35 and $40 billion in 1979, or about a quarter of the total amount expended on personal health care. Relman does not include in these figures the revenues of health services management consulting companies, attorneys, construction companies, continuing education, accounting services, or information services.

Organizational Differences

There are significant differences in how freestanding hospitals and multi-unit (five or more) hospital system corporations are organized, regardless of whether the multi-unit system is for-profit, not-for-profit, or public. Some of the key organizational differences are hypothesized in table 9, which has been adapted from Henry Mintzberg's categories of the professional bureaucracy (the freestanding hospital) and the divisionalized firm (the hospital in a multi-unit system).

As Mintzberg sees it, the key coordinating mechanisms in the freestanding hospital (the professional bureaucracy) are the standardized skills of the physicians; in the multi-unit hospital system (the divisionalized firm), the coordinating mechanisms are the standardized outputs or services. These outputs or services are subject to cost and quality controls under the direction of specialists at the central headquarters.

Dominant in the production process of the freestanding hospital is the operating core of attending physicians; dominant in the production process of the multi-unit hospital system are middle-level managers. There is much less formalized behavior and less planning and performance control in the freestanding hospital than in the multi-unit hospital system.

Table 9: Structural Dimensions of Freestanding Hospitals and Multi-Unit Hospital Systems*

Dimension	Professional Bureaucracy (Freestanding)	Divisionalized Firm (Multi-Unit)
Key coordinating mechanisms	Standardization of skills	Standardization of output
Key part of the organization	Operating core	Middle line
Formalization of behavior	Little (bureaucratic)	Much (bureaucratic)
Planning and control	Little	Much performance control
Strategic apex	External liaison Conflict resolution	Strategic portfolio Performance control
Middle line	Controlled by professionals: much mutual adjustment	Formulation of divisional strategy, managing operations
Power	Professionals	Middle line

*Adapted with permission from Henry Mintzberg. *The Structuring of Organizations* (Englewood Cliffs, N.J.: Prentice-Hall, ©1979), pp. 466–67.

Managerial Differences

Top managers in the freestanding hospital tend to focus on external liaison and conflict resolution. In a similar hospital in a multi-unit system, top managers are more concerned with controlling performance and with deciding lines of business and related financial and marketing strategies.

In the freestanding hospital, middle-level line managers tend to be controlled by physicians, although there is some mutual adjustment between physicians and managers. In hospitals in multi-unit corporations, these managers help formulate division strategy and manage operations more directly. Power accrues to the middle-level line managers rather than to physicians, as it does in freestanding hospitals.

There is some support in the health services management literature for Mintzberg's hypotheses. Harry Malm finds that, in the not-for-profit multi-unit hospital system, managers do not get involved in many of the details of accounting, reporting, and purchasing. Staff at central headquarters carries out independent reseach into construction, financing, new operational techniques, and business procedures. The local hospital manager is free, therefore, to focus upon the community and its health needs and to plan ways in which the hospital may better answer these needs.

I interpret this to mean that the local hospital manager adopts a marketing rather than a production orientation, while central headquarters determines performance standards and sets up control systems to hold the local manager accountable for production. Such a set-up is radically different from the more traditional "not operating at a loss and keeping the doctors happy."

David Springate and Melissa McNeil indicate that the following performance standards are set by central headquarters staff in for-profit multi-unit hospital systems: supplies on hand, amount of earnings, ratio of number of beds set up and staffed to number of patients, ratio of number of nurses to number of patients, and ratio of number of total personnel to number of patients. Managers are differentially rewarded, punished, and trained in these organizations according to whether they meet or surpass standards in these areas.

Richard Martin, who is now vice-president for operations of Health Group, a second generation for-profit multihospital corporation, and who has been a manager in freestanding not-for-profit (tax exempt) hospitals as well, contrasts managerial functions and responsibilities in the two kinds of hospitals.

Martin suggests that the chief executive of a freestanding not-for-profit hospital spends 20 to 35 percent of his or her time in meetings. There are more steps in the decision-making process, and the manager must allow more time to build a consensus. The manager must touch base monthly with all members of the executive committee of the governing board and must spend considerable time orienting new medical staff board members. He or she must continually cultivate people, plant seeds of ideas in their minds, make their ideas other people's ideas, and be subtle.

Board members of the medium-sized (300 beds) and smaller freestanding not-for-profit hospital tend to view board meetings as community service rather than business occasions, and they serve on the board primarily to gratify their egos or to fulfill their sense of mission, according to Martin. As competition increases among providers, Martin believes that progressive hospitals and particularly regional systems, will evolve to smaller (seven to ten) compensated boards of directors, selected for their business talent and value in capital formation under cost reimbursement.

Martin believes that boards and managers in these freestanding tax exempt hospitals often have a false sense of security. They are sitting "on a big pile of bricks" and they adopt a quasi-civil-service mentality. They behave as though they will get paid whether the hospital runs at 60 percent or 80 percent occupancy. Such hospitals are less willing to take risks, especially when the risks involve large expenditures. Their boards and managers "frequently lack experience with large credit lines, bond issues, and financial leverage."

Martin suggests that managers in for-profit multi-unit hospital corporations can make and implement decisions more quickly. Decisions in these hospitals are made primarily on the basis of return on investment or market share rather than politics or image. A defect of the for-profit perspective, according to Martin, is its short-term focus on this year's earning statement and incentive compensation, which can amount to 40 percent of a manager's base salary.

Martin suggests that goals tend to be more clear-cut in for-profit multi-unit hospital corporations. Managers in Health Group are rewarded on the basis of whether they attain the following goals:

—Targeted income, measured on a preinterest, premanagement fee, pretax basis

—Control of assets employed to budgeted levels (emphasis on accounts receivable management and capital budgeting)

—Marketing plan implementation

—Quality assurance program implementation

Advantages and Disadvantages for the Manager

Multi-unit hospital systems, regardless of their auspices, offer managers greater opportunities for upward mobility in the same organization. They offer excellent opportunities to learn because they have more sophisticated control systems and specialized functional expertise in many management areas. In for-profit multi-unit hospital corporations, financial rewards tend to be more tied to performance; they may be sizable, relative to the manager's base salary.

The disadvantages are characteristic of any large for-profit multi-unit corporation: upward mobility will require the manager to move to different areas of the country. Entry-level managers are replaceable and have little job security unless their performance quickly meets centrally set standards. Some of the for-profit chains are managed by promoters rather than by operations people and are driven by financial rather than service considerations. In the very large for-profit multi-unit hospital corporations, managers are constrained by corporate policies and standards. In hospitals in these corporations, managers may have difficulty in changing policies and standards quickly in order to respond to local operating constraints and opportunities. There are more managers in the large hospital corporations, and this can make for more complex intramanagerial politics and for many levels separating the new or younger manager and the top corporate decision makers.

VI
Managing Yourself

Our judgment is in great part what other people think it is.

Ray Brown

One mistake that is made in confrontation situations where there are complex issues and legitimate differences in opinion is to take opposing opinions personally.

Norman Urmy

What the manager has most control over in working with subordinates, colleagues, allies, and others is himself or herself. In this chapter I discuss how aspects of the four managerial role sets discussed in Chapter 2— scanning the environment, negotiating the political terrain, motivating others, and generating and allocating resources—are related to one's development as a manager. I present examples to illustrate.

Keeping informed, earning trust, understanding values, and making decisions are aspects of managerial behavior that correspond closely to the four role sets referred to above. This correspondence is shown in table 10. Certain aspects of managerial behavior, such as keeping informed, cut across role sets. Also cutting across role sets are other ways of viewing managerial performance that are discussed in this chapter: managing time and presence, managing yourself with others, and managing yourself with your boss.

Keeping Informed

EXAMPLE:

Claire Rogers, director of nursing at Highsmith Teaching Hospital, wishes to improve the productivity of the nursing department, yet there is no clear-cut logic as to which items are charged against nursing accounts and which are charged against other departments' accounts. There has been no calculation of the financing needed to allow replacement employees to be hired and trained before old employees leave. Rogers has no way of predicting which charges are made directly to the patient and which to the nursing unit. She is unable to predict what new major equipment may come on the market for the next fiscal year. Rogers has not been able to determine what data the hospital collects on nursing performance and how these data are aggregated and analyzed. Using the data that she has, Rogers can make nursing productivity look either rosy or dismal, depending on how costs and revenues are allocated and what standards are used for comparison. Clearly, to do the job asked of her, Rogers has to see developed a data system that can give her the answers she needs.

Table 10: Role Sets and Aspects of
Managerial Behavior

Role Set	Aspect of Managerial Behavior
Scanning the environment	Keeping informed
Negotiating the political terrain	Earning trust
Motivating others	Understanding values
Generating and allocating resources	Making decisions

One of the key advantages you have as a manager is your access to and control of information. By virtue of your position, certain information flows regularly to you. For example, hospital administrators regularly receive, from state and national hospital associations and from governmental agencies, information about local, state, and national regulations affecting hospitals and advice on how to comply with or adapt to these regulations. Much internal communication must go through a manager's office before it is distributed throughout the organization. Managers often have to approve expenditure requests, new personnel slots, the amounts and methods of remuneration to employees and contractors, the allocation of space, and the design and timing of the organization's long-range planning process. Thus anyone who wants organizational resources is likely to seek support or tolerance from management before making a serious formal claim.

Important requirements of your job may be to help the organization (or a department in it) adapt to environmental pressures and opportunities and to coordinate the activities of different groups and departments in order to attain organizational goals. Appropriate decisions in these areas depend upon accurate, timely, and shared information and upon a fair and workable decision-making process.

You should have sufficient time and staff assistance to find out how other organizations respond to problems and to develop information systems that will generate the data needed in decision making. You may want to know what kinds of services organizations similar to yours are initiating or closing out. What are industry-wide standards regarding cost per unit of service, collection ratios, average days in accounts payable and receivable, and reimbursement rates? How do other organizations prepare to comply with new or existing regulations? How are your peers remunerated and evaluated? How do organizations similar to yours recruit physicians and key employees? What kinds of complaints do their patients make most frequently? What are the most important complaints their patients make? How do other managers respond to such complaints? How do community groups view your organization and the services it provides? The list is endless, and you can acquire more information than you can process effectively. Therefore you must structure the flow of information: get only the information you need; avoid information that can be adequately processed by others.

Some managers may not know what information is available within their own organizations or even within their own files. Despite a cluttered office and piles of papers on desks and tables, they say they know "where everything is," or they claim this knowledge on behalf of their secretaries. The information they require may, however, be "in the files," and finding it may take so long that by the time they or their secretaries have located it, the need for it has passed. Other managers, with neat offices and bare desk tops, claim to throw out everything that is not necessary and to need nothing that they have ever thrown out. For some of them, this is actually true.

Some good rules about information for a new manager are (1) always make a copy of any important memo or document you are sending to someone else, in case he or she misplaces it; (2) number all the pages in your memos so that when a point is discussed everyone can find it; (3) make memos self-contained, so that readers do not need other documents in order to understand your key points; (4) do not use abbreviations without having first spelled them out.

You must decide what you need to know in order to carry out managerial performance requirements. Consider the basis upon which you are being evaluated and by whom. What kind of documentation must you marshall to persuade those who are evaluating you that you are doing an adequate job? What information will help convince them that you are making an essential contribution? No one should perceive you as so unsatisfactory that they remove you from their sphere of interest or from the organization's.

You also require information about your political situation. This information is not usually expressed in statistics, but it can be elicited in conversations with persons in the controlling coalition (see Chapter 10). You need information about who your allies and opponents are before issues are discussed in open meetings.

Given limited time and energy, you must focus your information gathering on important problems or opportunities that you can sometimes affect. To do this, you must learn to differentiate among matters that are unimportant, matters that are important but that you can do little or nothing about, and matters that are important and that you *can* do something about within a short time.

A common error of new managers is to define as unimportant something that members of the controlling coalition define as important. A second error is to devote an inordinate amount of attention to problems that the organization cannot solve or is not ready to solve, for political or other reasons. This does not mean that you should not gather information about such problems: this should be done if only to remind people that there is an important problem about which the organization has some information but which it is not ready to act upon yet.

Obtain whatever useful information you can that is available at little or no cost. Remember, obtaining other needed information may cost more time, money, or political capital than it is worth to you personally.

Earning Trust

EXAMPLE:

Stan Lewis, marketing director of Urban HMO, meets regularly with Jon Warner and Gloria Lopez, president and vice-president of the HMO's community advisory board. Lopez complains about discrimination against Hispanic workers and patients and wants the community board to have the final say about HMO budget decisions. Lewis explains that the community board is advisory and that neither the Department of Health and Human Services nor the city government, both of which fund the HMO, requires the type of community participation that Lopez wants. Lewis adds that any complaint made by Lopez or Warner will be looked into and the results explained to the community board. The community board can discuss all budget items; their comments will be forwarded to the funding agencies, but final budget decisions will be made by HMO management.

Here is a situation in which there is conflict of interest between the perceptions and perhaps even the goals of advisory council members and HMO management. Lopez, a former worker in the HMO, seeks jobs and dignity for Hispanic workers, some of whom are her friends. Lewis, the marketing director and assistant administrator, may not earn her trust, but he can convince her that he is honest. From Lewis' point of view, some of Lopez' friends may be good workers, and some of her complaints may be justified. Progress may be made, therefore, in accommodating each other's goals. Even if Lewis and Lopez dislike one another, they may, over time, respect the hard work and competence that each brings to the bargaining table.

If a large part of managerial success or avoidance of failure depends upon others' trusting you, how are you to earn and build this trust? It is easier to gain people's trust to begin with than to regain it after you have lost it. Trust can only be earned over time, as others see your behavior, monitor your decisions, and judge whether you are taking their values into account as you behave, decide, and implement decisions. They will also be evaluating how predictable you are in what you say and do.

Many persons have reason to distrust any new manager even before the manager has joined the organization. There are many possible reasons for this. Such persons may not have been doing their jobs. They may have been obtaining more organizational resources for themselves at less cost than you will think is appropriate. They may have been doing a good job, but in the course of it may have incurred the enmity of important persons in the organization who they fear will use you to diminish their roles and power.

Managers with whom you work want to feel that their contribution is being rewarded fairly in relation to yours. Even more important than absolutes can be relative pay, benefits, and privileges. Co-workers have strong feelings about the recognition they get in relation to the contribution they make or the pressures they have to withstand. Therefore you must be careful in what you say and how you act in front of them. Managers at your level may fear you more than do persons on a level below you. They may feel they are competing with you rather than working on the same managerial team. You may feel the same way. Conflicts of interest between you and other managers are real, because you are competing for status, recognition, and whatever higher-level positions may be available.

Critical to earning the trust of subordinates is their perception of you as fair. This means that they see you as taking into proper account their opinions and interests. They want you to consult them before you form an opinion about them or make decisions that affect them. To the extent that subordinates fear you, they are not likely to share with you all their reasons for backing or opposing certain policies. At the same time, subordinates are likely to insist that you do what you said you would do when this is consistent with their interests.

Your superiors are unlikely to fear you. They may be more afraid that they will make a wrong policy decision because they are relying on you and have lacked the time, the will, or the judgment to be adequately informed about the matter. In making policy decisions, many superiors seek to follow the leadership of someone reliable whom they trust. Usually these people are the managers whom they have selected and who are dependent upon them for their positions and remuneration. Try within reasonable bounds to please your superiors. You will lose the trust of superiors through incompetence or by arousing the enmity of physicians, with whom they must also work. Other ways to lose the trust of others, according to Griffith, are lack of candor, confusion of values, unprofessional behavior, erratic behavior, and lack of preparation.

It is important, perhaps more so for the organization than for you, that you earn the trust of community and employee leaders. You should be careful what you say to such representatives and officials; otherwise, in conflict situations they may seek to mobilize people on the basis of personal antagonism toward you or to exercise claims on the organization based on what they say you told them.

It is helpful to meet with community and employee leaders before urgent problems arise, in order to learn their views as to how the goals and behavior of your organization effect their members. It is useful in such meetings for you to explain organizational views of the responsibilities and behavior of their groups. This helps establish the perception that both sides have similar concerns. Both sides usually "get more" from each other by trusting each other than by acting as adversaries. Managers can and should make demands of community and employee groups rather than always being on the defensive. Such demands range from requesting complaints and suggestions about improving services to requesting volunteers and donations.

It is important for you to review with such groups what they see as important problems and to explain carefully and in detail why certain demands can or cannot be met and why further information is needed in certain areas. Such review meetings require time to prepare for and to conduct, but they often have positive benefits for you and your organization. Certain requests from community and employee groups can be met at little cost. By meeting with you, groups may come to understand organizational constraints of which they were not previously aware. Individuals on each side can get to know each other better, thus building, it is hoped, a reserve of trust that will alleviate some of the anger and bitterness of possible future confrontations. There is nothing wrong with mutually acknowledging conflict. In fact, denying that conflict of interest exists may build false expectations as to what key participants on each side can reasonably expect from each other.

EXAMPLE:
Wyatt Burns, the vice-president for planning and support services for Urban HMO, does not understand why two of his subordinates, Kim Greenhut and Bruce Wright, have been promoted to presidencies of Second Urban HMO and Suburban HMO, which with Urban HMO are subsidiary organizations of Grand Alliance HMO, a national system serving four million members.

Burns has been with the Urban HMO for 20 years and is acknowledged as expert, brainy, energetic, and productive. Tim McGregor, formerly president of Urban HMO and now president of Grand Alliance HMO, has told Burns that he is as highly paid and esteemed in his present position as are the persons formerly his subordinates and now presidents in the other plans, and that the reason Burns was not offered one of the presidential jobs is because of his lack of line experience. Kim Greenhut commented subsequently to Burns that the real reason Burns did not get the promotion was because McGregor feels that Burns is unpredictable in his loyalty to the organization, that McGregor does not feel as safe with Burns as with Wright or herself.

Greenhut added that she had not heard this from McGregor herself, it is only her supposition.

The reader may ask what benefit there might be for Burns to better understand the differences between his own values and those of McGregor. A partial answer is that (a) Burns might have changed some of his behavior if he had realized the value attached by McGregor to company loyalty; and (b) Burns might have been less frustrated by McGregor's promotion decisions if he had better understood the real as opposed to the stated reasons for McGregor's actions.

Understanding Values

Some organizations promote only from within. Some believe that there is such a thing as an "organizational personality" and that anyone who cannot adjust to the way things are done in that organization should go elsewhere. Certain physicians and trustees feel uncomfortable working for or with persons from minority groups, Ivy Leaguers, or physically handicapped persons; is anybody going to do anything about their not hiring or supporting such persons? What are the values regarding such issues in your organization and among those upon whose approval you depend for job security and financial remuneration?

You are categorized by your skin color, ethnic group, religion, age, sex, and education; most of these factors you cannot change. Some people may resent you *because* you belong to the same group they do, viewing you as a rival or as a source of vulnerability: if you fail, they may be perceived as failures too. On the other hand, a majority of persons in the same ethnic, age, or religious group to which you belong may feel more comfortable working with you. Such group membership may help you perform effectively. You are also categorized by your dress, appearance, manners, and reaction under pressure; some of these factors you can change.

Employees may feel that you regard them primarily as cogs in an organizational machine. Do you value them or appear to value them only in terms of their contribution to organizational effectiveness? Most people want others with whom they work closely to value them as human beings, regardless of their contribution to organizational effectiveness. Lack of contribution may not be their fault. Even if it is, they may have been willing to change during the first years of their employment, but their superiors did not help them to change. If your employees feel that you do not value them as persons, their performance may worsen, and you will be unable to do anything about it at a cost acceptable to you.

Your values and those of top management in your organization *do* affect your chances for success and job security. It is not uncommon for important persons in an organization to say the opposite of what they mean or to be purposely vague in order to test a young manager. You must walk a fine line between being true to yourself and pleasing important people in the organization whose cooperation—or at least lack of active opposition—you need to effectively carry out your responsibilities. Some managers do not have to walk this line: they view themselves and others as instruments for achieving their bosses' objectives. Many bosses do not care what your values are as long as you do what they want and your work is acceptable.

Most of us managers cannot view ourselves as mere instruments: it goes against our ethics and our training. Top management changes and the values of its members often conflict. Managers are paid to work things out somehow, to arbitrate between parties—in Norman Urmy's words, to get "consensus by juggling things simultaneously and dealing with diverse, competing interest groups across a broad spectrum of skills and educational backgrounds."

The danger you face in always being true to yourself or to your values is, of course, that important others may disagree with your view, even when you are motivated primarily by organizational rather than by personal considerations. Then, if you persist too strongly, they may object to you personally to an extent that can compromise your actual and potential contributions to organizational effectiveness. This can happen even if you are "right" in organizational terms.

Sometimes, when your values conflict with those of powerful others, you must decide how much to fight for a policy and whether a policy difference is worth leaving the organization. Consider that the organizaton may be better off if you do leave. Consider also how secure your job may be, relative to other job options, should you persist in working actively against present policy and those who have determined it. Consider changing your opinions.

There is something to be said in theory for having managers around who generally disagree with the main tendency of those in power, but top management is seldom sufficiently broadminded or rich in resources for such a luxury. One reason for having such independent managers on staff is to provide top managers with important objections to policy decisions before they are made, in order to assure effective implementation. Such managers may also be helpful in long-range planning, assuming they are sensitive to changing environmental pressures or to past strategies that, although discarded, may be useful in the future.

There are advantages in working only with persons whom you have selected and with whom you feel comfortable. If you are newly appointed and want substantial change, and if you are willing to pay the price in human suffering to accomplish this, firing many of the incumbents may considerably increase the contribution of a managerial work force over two or three years. If nothing else, you may need to rely absolutely on your employees for minimum standards of performance, as you define them, and for absolute loyalty in the political infighting that can be so much a part of organizational life.

There is also something to be said for rewarding past loyalty and past productivity when a manager's present contribution is less than it should be. This does not require, I believe, continuation of present salary and other perquisites. Usually in such cases, rather than changing both pay and responsibilities, attempts are first made to "rehabilitate" the manager and then to influence him or her to seek early retirement. Of course, many managers may resist lower salary and perquisites, even if they would enhance productivity.

There is seldom a right or wrong that can be objectively established among managers when values clash. There is behavior that works or does not work over the short- or long-term in the perception of a top management that itself changes continuously in composition and in intensity of feelings. What is important is that you know your own values, know how they differ from those of your employer or of significant others, and take these differences into consideration before you act. Obviously, you should consider differences in values before taking a job. If you have strong feelings against profits in health care or against managers who are secretive and who dislike participative management, do not work for those organizations or those managers. What is difficult is deciding what to do when you have become aware of such important value differences only after you have already been employed.

Making Decisions

EXAMPLE:

Dr. Lisle Kent, the president of the medical staff of Glory Hospital, has advised Victor Alan, the new hospital administrator, that he is ill-advised to pressure the medical staff to agree to a new risk management program. First, there must be other things Alan can do as hospital administrator that are important and less distasteful to the medical staff. Second, the lawyers whom Alan wants to conduct the risk management program are the prosecuting attorneys for malpractice cases in another state, and their written guarantee not to prosecute Glory Hospital's physicians will not sufficiently alleviate the physicians' fears. Because of several recent malpractice losses for the hospital, Alan insists on having the lawyers make a presentation to the hospital medical staff. The medical staff votes down Alan's program.

Why did Alan make what seems to be such a wrong decision? Was it because he is stupid, did not think things through, failed to check his ideas out in advance with sufficient numbers of the medical staff, lacked experience, or all of the above? Or was his a right decision, the opposing of which will result in more malpractice at Glory Hospital? Alan justifies his action by his concern for patient care, but how are physicians going to perceive such an action? Is this a values issue, a decision issue, or both? I believe it is both.

Managers may judge problems to be more serious than they are, recommend unnecessary action, and generate unnecessary conflict, or they may underrate the importance of serious problems and fail to respond soon enough. There are very few situations that require immediate action by the health services manager, but those that do will result in serious consequences if no decision, or an inappropriate decision, is made. In such cases, you cannot waste time debating what to do next or whom to call. Disaster, fire, imminent threat of malpractice, and strike are situations in which the timing of your decision is vital. You should have a prepared repertoire of responses for emergencies that are likely to occur.

It may be difficult to differentiate on the spot an emergency from an urgent situation. You cannot predict when a specific type of emergency is likely to occur, but you can learn what situations require immediate action and you can predict what types of emergencies you are likely to face. Your actions as a manager in responding to emergencies that occur in your first few years in an organization may be critical to your continued effectiveness or your survival in the job.

Review continuously and carefully what it is that you are being paid to do. Was Alan (see the example) being paid primarily to get along with the hospital medical staff (and was this made clear to him, or did he seek to make it clear, or wasn't it obvious?) or to protect patients from avoidable malpractice? In the values clash would Alan have made a wiser decision by establishing an effective risk management program in some other way, such as by consulting with the state hospital association? Would he antagonize the medical staff by contacting the state hospital association? Would the state hospital association program be sufficiently thorough? Does it matter?

One alternative that managers can choose is deciding not to decide. New managers often err by making too many decisions rather than too few. According to Chester Barnard, "the fine art of executive decision consists in not deciding questions that are not now pertinent, in not deciding prematurely, in not making decisions that cannot be made effective, and in not making decisions that others should make."

As Urmy points out in Chapter 10, health services managers do not spend most of their time making organizational decisions. The basic resource at your disposal is yourself—who you are and what you say. The decisions that you do make are often embarrassingly small ones in view of some of your managerial expectations—what to say to nurse X or doctor Y and when and where to say it. Therefore, think before you speak, keep informed, work on understanding others' values, and do your homework before recommending controversial action.

Managing Time and Presence

The cost of managing your time can be minimal relative to the benefits. Some health services organizations function all 8,760 hours of the year, assuming a 365-day year. You may work as much as 12 hours a day for 5½ days a week, take two weeks vacation and seven holidays a year, and yet not be regarded by most Americans as working too hard. You may work as little as seven hours a day for five days a week, take a month's vacation and 12 holidays a year, and yet not be regarded as working too little by many of the same people. Thus, ignoring sick time, the acceptable variance in your work time as a manager may be as many as 1,659 hours per year, or a ratio of over 2:1—quite a difference. Who is to say that the person who works twice as many hours contributes twice as much, or even any more, to organizational effectiveness? On the other hand, it is difficult to argue with the proposition that, generally speaking, one person working twice as many hours as another will accomplish or contribute more.

Getting people to work longer hours can contribute to organizational effectiveness, assuming that the quantity and quality of their work during regular hours does not diminish to offset the additional hours worked. You should decide how many hours and days you want to work. Managers as well as other employees conduct personal business during working hours. This includes making appointments with their physicians and reading the newspapers, both of which can be considered work-related. As long as you are in your office or on the premises, you are available for phone calls relating to work or to respond to a work emergency. By conducting personal affairs while being easily available, you are actually working for the organizaton, at least on an on-call basis.

Many managers spend long hours working at home, especially doing paperwork. There may be fewer interruptions at home and therefore they can accomplish more in a given amount of time. Others make work-related phone calls after hours for the same reason. A former colleague of mine started a second work day at 9 p.m. each evening, working until 2 a.m. and then awakening the next morning at 7 a.m. This man was always relaxed and gracious in his office and people wondered how he accomplished so much.

Given that you are working a certain number of hours, the next question is what activities you should spend most of your time on. To a large extent, this question will be decided for you by others: there are always meetings you have to attend and people you have to speak with inside and outside the organization. Some managers are able to do two things at once, for example making lists of things to do or reading their mail while attending meetings. Others are able to go to meetings late and to leave them early.

Analyze how you spend your time (say for a two-week period) so that you can better understand your work patterns. Then you can decide which activities you want or need to spend more or less time on. You need to schedule some uninterrupted blocks of time during the week or month for important planning and other creative work. You need to reserve uninterrupted time as well for those who are accountable to you and for your superiors and peers, time that is not spent responding to crises but anticipating problems, implementing policy decisions, and earning trust.

Ross Webber suggests the following tactics for managing your time: insulating yourself from incoming communications; isolating yourself or withdrawing physically, so interruptions are eliminated except in emergencies; grouping responses to others, such as returning phone calls; and delegating or discontinuing certain responses.

Webber cautions that the manager should not attempt to minimize available time which is used for response, which he feels should make up more than half the manager's time. Moreover, he recommends that managers "be open, patient, and truly responsive" during response time.

As a manager, you need to manage your presence as well as your time. You need to be present in others' work areas, where they feel more comfortable, and to observe first hand how services are being provided by your organization in various departments and units.

Off-the-job presence can be important as well. Workers may view you differently after interacting with you in situations where your status is more nearly equal. Occasions for interaction may include shopping at the supermarket, working out at the gym, being a physician's patient, or attending Parent-Teacher Association meetings with a subordinate. Of course, others may view you more or less positively as a result of such interaction, depending on your behavior. William Ouchi suggests that it may be beneficial to interact with subordinates in situations where status is reversed, that managers and subordinates tend to trust each other more and to empathize with each other more as a result.

There are no set rules for how much time you should spend in different locations. It takes a great deal of time and effort to visit people and to respond to their concerns and suggestions. One value of analyzing where and how you spend your time is that it shows you what you are actually doing. Without such information, it is difficult to manage your time.

<u>Your Relationship with Others</u>

EXAMPLE:
Bill Jones, department head in inhalation therapy at Glory Hospital, wants a
raise. Victor Alan, the hospital administrator, feels that Jones is being paid
fairly relative to other department heads as well as to other inhalation therapy
heads in ten neighboring hospitals. Dr. Tony Ricardo, chief of pulmonary
medicine and vice-president of the medical staff, argues that Jones should be
paid ten percent more than he is making: Jones, he says, is "that good," he
may leave, and the department is highly profitable.

An effective managerial style will not solve the problem of inequities
in salaries—and the decision about the raise is Alan's; he cannot effectively
buck it on to anyone else.

If Alan decides not to give Jones a raise, he can say that Jones'
request is out of line with current policy and that sufficient cause has not
been shown for an exception to be made. Jones has been given the maximum raise for department heads this year. But Alan must still consider
whether and how to respond to Jones' arguments that inhalation therapists
at two similar hospitals in the state make more than he does and that his
salary was too low when he accepted the position initially. Alan may think
that Jones is relying too much on Dr. Ricardo's leverage and resent such
interference with managerial prerogatives.

Should Alan explain his position to Jones in Alan's office or in a
pleasant restaurant? How long should the interview take? How patient
should Alan be with Jones in listening to him repeat his arguments? How
does Alan respond when Jones says he might have to seek a job elsewhere?
Does Alan say, "Well, Jones, that's your decision and it would be a great
loss to the hospital"? Or does he say, "That's your decision, Bill; there's
nothing I can do to compel you to continue working here, but we sure need
you a lot"?

What, if anything, does Alan say to Dr. Ricardo? Where should Alan
discuss the Jones situation with Ricardo? For how long should Alan discuss
it with him? How responsive should Alan be to Ricardo's dependence upon
Jones, even if Alan thinks Ricardo can get someone else who is adequate
for less money? Should Alan talk to Ricardo before he talks to Jones, and
should he touch base as well with Mr. Strong, the trustee chairman of the
finance committee?

Does anyone really care how you manage, as long as you get the job
done? Can you actually change your management style? Many managers are
not conscious of how they do what they do: What works, works; what
doesn't work, doesn't. You may not be able to separate style from content.
When urged to change your style, you may respond, "I can't be someone

I'm not. If something isn't working, it's as much somebody else's fault as it is mine. If it is my fault, maybe I am in the wrong job."

Aspects of managerial style have been discussed in the section on Persona, in Chapter 2. Managers can control, to some degree, their appearance and work habits. Managerial style is important in any job, although in some jobs it is not crucial to effectiveness. An inappropriate style can make managing more difficult and less pleasant than it need be. Is your managerial style congruent with those whom you must influence? This is an important question, because persuading others is an important part of most managerial jobs. Your style must be comfortable for you, and it must be perceived by others as authentic, otherwise you will be seen as trying to be someone or something you are not.

Others may be looking for signals from you to confirm what they think you are really like, how you really think. You may want to conceal or to flaunt your feelings and biases. No matter how you respond to others, or how your secretary responds, or what your stationary looks like, or how large your office is, these aspects of your persona are going to be weighed and interpreted by others. You need to take into account how others are going to view your choices in these areas. Remember that few people, if any, will tell you when your style is offensive to them or to others.

My advice to the entry-level manager is to work long hours, dress conservatively, and be a responsive listener. These activities are likely to be perceived as valuable, at least officially, by those physicians and trustees upon whom you are most dependent. Of course, managers, like everyone else, are persons first and managers second. Your managerial behavior and style should be consonant with your personal values and the values of those whom you love. You may be surprised, however, at what changes you can make in your managerial style without conflicting with your personal values.

When you make substantial policy changes, you may want to give participants no reason other than the policy itself for disliking you. Like political candidates, you do not want key groups to dislike you. Of course, avoiding controversy may cause some people to view you as evasive, indirect, and passive. This might be a lesser risk, especially in organizations where the manager's role, in terms of coodinating and integrating the medical care production process, has not yet been fully accepted among physicians.

Managers do not or cannot always check out their decisions, or ways of implementing their decisions, with persons who claim they should have been consulted. Reasons for this include time pressures, laziness, and the difficulty of explaining a complicated matter to a physician whom you see only in passing in the hall or whom you can reach only by telephone. Managers may sometimes touch base officially with department heads or trustees only after responding to a fleeting conversation initiated by someone else about items on other agendas. A trustee may assent to some decision without fully grasping the implications behind it because he or she is more concerned at this moment about a spouse's health, his or her own business, or other matters.

It is commonly believed that lack of communication is the reason that people who work in the same organization do not get along with, distrust, or intensely dislike each other. This is only partly true. People see what they want to see, hear what they want to hear. What people see and hear may not be at all what you are actually doing or saying, let alone what you intend to do or say.

Much personal conflict is rooted in conflicting values or interests; poor communication is a symptom of the conflict and contributes to it. Conflicting values or interests can cause people to dislike or fear each other. Personal dislike does not have to interfere with work relations unless the persons' jobs are interdependent. It is typically this interdependency that deepens personal dislike and fear.

Part of your job as a manager is to mediate conflict among others, whether they are subordinates, peers, or superiors. Another part of your job is to deal with any of your own internal conflicts that affect making and implementing managerial decisions.

It is essential that you manage yourself in such a way that you do not unintentionally magnify conflict. You want conflicting persons to increasingly trust you, or at least not to distrust you, so that mutual accommodations can be made over disputed matters. You may keep telling them, "We are on the same team and must work together," whereas they may keep saying, "We may be on the same team, but I don't pay the same costs or reap the same benefits that you do according to my contributions, qualifications, or needs." You may be thinking, "I know, but my situation is even worse regarding my costs and benefits relative to other participants in this organization." They may be thinking, "You're the manager, and you can do something about my case. This is the job you are being paid to do, to alleviate the worst forms of inequity." If you say what you are thinking, either or both of you may lack the time and will to continue the dialogue.

Some managers may attempt to convince claimants that (1) getting them their equitable share is not the job that the manager is being paid to do—rather, the manager is being paid to prevent the organization from operating at a loss and to minimize discontent among the medical staff; (2) theirs is not one of the worst cases of inequity in the organization; (3) the organization is not willing to pay whatever amount it takes to retain a given level of contribution from them or from anyone else; and (4) the perception of what benefits and costs are appropriate for each member of the organization will vary depending upon which member you ask. This perception will also vary with the claimants' current and expected contributions to the organization. Moreover, the perceived magnitude of these contributions also varies depending upon whom you ask and how you ask them.

Talking to claimants in this way is not likely to calm them. Logical or not, such a rationalistic, formal style is inappropriate to most conflict situations. The point I wish to make is that managers must manage themselves during such confrontations. Get the other persons to talk. Do not take what others say personally, even if they are being personal. This does not mean that you have to put up with personal abuse, only that you should not respond in kind. Prepare yourself for such meetings in advance. What arguments are claimants likely to raise and how are you going to respond? Do you have the facts to back up your arguments? What are the available facts? How are claimants going to respond to your arguments, reasons, and expectations? If they are likely to respond negatively, how can you, by means of your managerial style, soften the impact, not lose their trust, and gain their respect, even though they differ with you as to a particular decision?

Your Relationship With Your Boss

EXAMPLE:

Lou Baines has been working for five years as assistant administrator at Highsmith Hospital, and he believes he deserves a raise. True, Baines has gotten a cost-of-living increase each year, but he feels now that his entry salary was too low. Baines and his wife Betty have two children. Baines works very hard. People like him and tell him when he asks for a raise that he deserves it. Ned Wainwright, Baines' superior, sees what Baines is talking about as an exceptions policy. Everyone else gets or does not get a raise every year according to established procedures. Why should Baines be any different? Wainwright is constrained in responding to Baines' claims by organizational and personal considerations. With whom does Wainwright have to get Baines' raise cleared? Does Wainwright feel that he himself is fairly paid? How will other managers react if Baines' request is granted?

What is Baines prepared to do if he does not get a raise? Is getting a raise really so important? The amount of money Baines makes is important for obvious reasons: it determines his spending and saving; it is a mark of his worth and status; and it can help or hinder him in getting another job. However, if Baines only keeps $1,000 of a $2,000 raise because of taxes how much additional saving and spending can he do on $20 a week?

Should Baines really worry a lot about what other managers make? It may not be fair if they make more than Baines does, relative to their contribution, but Baines may make trouble for himself by insisting upon fairness. Insisting is perfectly appropriate if Baines is willing to pay the price for attempting to obtain equity, regardless of whether he actually achieves it.

If Lou Baines decides that he really needs more money, his best strategy may be to obtain a position in another organization. If he cannot obtain such a position now, he must work harder and more effectively, so that he will be able to obtain such a position in the future. What Baines should not do is jeopardize his current position by pushing too hard for more money. Pushing for a raise is not always viewed favorably, especially by some employers who believe that their not-for-profit organization should be subsidized by employees.

Perhaps Baines should give equal attention to the expense side of his financial equation. Is he knowledgeable about deductible expenses? Baines should take every tax deduction he can and document them adequately. Perhaps he should consider putting his family on a budget and analyzing variances from that budget and current patterns of expenditure. Baines should save and invest wisely. He should apply the good management he is supposedly doing at work to his family's financial planning.

Wainwright does not necessarily view Baines' request negatively. Baines is asking to be rewarded for superior performance. Does Wainwright agree that Baines's performance is superior? If so, does the organization wish to reward such performance or does it not? If not, Baines may continue to perform above the standards or he may not. If, however, Baines persists in asking for an "exceptional" raise after Wainwright has already explained why an exception cannot be made, Wainwright will view Baines' persistence negatively. If Wainwright wants to give Baines a raise anyway, adequate documentation is relatively easy to develop. If Wainwright wishes to treat Baines' request bureaucratically, Baines may wish to obtain the help of the personnel department in determining what types of reclassification are possible. If Wainwright is against giving Baines a raise, Baines is probably wasting his time in developing documentation.

It is easy to suggest to Baines that the time to negotiate pay and benefits was when he was first hired. But Baines may have wanted the position or the promotion so badly then that he would have taken any pay or benefits Wainwright might have given him in order to get the job.

Requesting a raise is an example of your having to manage yourself in relationship to your boss. I will examine now in more general terms what bosses and managers expect from each other and why their expectations of each other are not always met.

What the Boss Expects

The boss expects the manager to do what the manager says he or she will do unless circumstances dictate a change in plan. Any important change should be cleared in advance. The boss also expects a certain level of managerial contribution. This may be specified in terms of changes in performance of the departments or units the manager supervises. Changes in such performance may be expressed in terms of increased revenues, increased volume of services, or in decreased unit costs. A certain level of personal performance is expected as well. This may be specified qualitatively, for example by assessing how well the manager conducts meetings with community groups or how well the manager performs, and communicates the results of, staff work on special projects.

The boss wants to know how to help the manager accomplish the goals the manager has said he or she will accomplish. The boss wants no surprises: he or she wants to hear any bad news accurately and sufficiently in advance to respond adequately and calmly.

The boss wants loyalty. How can the boss be expected to protect the manager, especially when the manager has made a mistake, if the manager is not loyal? The loyal manager thinks about how some action or decision will affect the boss and the boss's position personally. The loyal manager tells the boss in advance when he or she thinks the boss is wrong and backs the boss wholeheartedly after the boss has made a decision, regardless of what it is.

The boss would like the manager to be cheerful and to take himself or herself seriously, but not too seriously. The boss has enough problems without having to worry about the manager's mental health. The boss's position demands respect and courtesy, which is the least the manager can give the person who is primarily responsible for determining whether the manager keeps his or her position, what the manager's working conditions are, and what the manager is and will be paid.

The boss expects political savvy. The manager is not to tell others that he or she is implementing a decision because the boss said to; rather, the manager is to explain to them the reasons for the decision. If the manager cannot readily think of some good and sufficient reasons, he or she should ask others why they are opposed to the policy and tell them that he or she will discuss their views with the boss. The manager may or may not attempt to pick apart their reasoning on the spot, depending on the cogency of their arguments, local political conditions, or the unevenness of the opponents' and the manager's respective statuses.

What the Manager Expects

The manager expects the boss to explain what is expected, what important job requirements are, and how and when work must be completed. If put in writing, there will be less misunderstanding as to what is expected. The manager should not agree to something he or she is not likely to complete by the expected time and at the expected level of excellence. The manager expects to be given sufficient autonomy to accomplish important requirements of his or her position. The manager should not be hampered by having to check back for approval of every action. The autonomy of new managers should be limited at first, until they understand the political environment and until the boss feels comfortable delegating authority to them. The manager expects to be rewarded adequately and fairly, relative to peers, for his or her contributions.

All workers have a right to be evaluated. This does not mean that a manager cannot be fired after receiving excellent evaluations, but regular evaluations are a matter of record and must be taken into account even by those who want to fire a manager. The manager cannot be expected to change his or her behavior unless the boss explains what the manager is doing wrong. To do the job effectively, the manager should be told regularly how his or her work fits into the wider frame of reference of managerial effort in the organization; otherwise, some events will be incomprehensible to the manager. Further, the manager may not be as helpful to the boss as he or she should be.

Just as the boss expects loyalty from the manager, the manager should expect the boss to protect him or her. The manager is going to make mistakes, and the boss must protect the manager in order to maintain the manager's effectiveness and energetic contribution to organizational objectives.

The manager expects the boss to show some consideration for the manager as an individual. If a manager has worked 16 hours a day for several weeks during labor negotiations, the boss should suggest that the manager take some time off. Before asking a manager to undertake a difficult or delicate assignment, the boss should ask the manager for his or her opinions and feelings so that both can consider whether or not the manager should take the assignment on, what strategy the manager should follow, and how the manager can best conduct himself or herself.

Why the Boss Does Not Get
The Expected Managerial Performance

The manager's behavior must meet minimum performance requirements; otherwise the boss will try to get rid of the manager, the manager will seek another job, or both. One reason a manager may not be able to perform agreed-upon tasks is that the tasks were unrealistic to begin with and neither boss nor manager realized it at the time. In such a situation the manager may be afraid to renegotiate what had been agreed to, hoping that the boss will see things now as the manager sees them, that the boss will forget, or that the manager can counterbalance low performance on one set of criteria with high performance on another.

The manager may have failed to tell the boss about constraints against the manager's making the expected contribution, about conflicting demands being made upon the manager's time by other important members of the organization, or about conflicting demands being made on the manager by members of his or her family. The boss may see the manager as lacking certain skills or beliefs because of inconsistencies in the boss's expectations. The manager may be afraid to ask the boss for help because it would make the manager look ignorant or because the manager does not want to be dependent on anyone.

It may take time for a boss to supervise a manager effectively. Perhaps the boss thinks the manager should be adequately motivated and trained not to need supervision; the manager may not agree. Perhaps the manager feels superior to the boss. The manager may be better trained and have more knowledge about operations than the boss does, yet the boss overrules the manager's recommendations on the basis of political considerations that may or may not be valid. Perhaps the boss does not like the manager as an individual. Perhaps the manager wants to blame the boss for his or her own mistakes. Perhaps the manager is insecure or working under pressures that are not related to the job.

Sometimes events occur so quickly that the manager does not have time to warn the boss. The bad news may be inaccurate, and the manager may lack the time or skills to validate it before informing the boss. Perhaps the physicians want to get rid of the boss; if the manager stands up and defends the boss, the physicians will want to get rid of the manager too. Perhaps certain physicians are more powerful than the boss and the manager's livelihood may depend upon not keeping the boss adequately informed or not implementing vigorously the boss's policies.

Cheerfulness, a sense of humor, and respect are hard to manufacture. Certain bosses may not favor excessive cheerfulness, humor, or deference anyway. As for political savvy, most managers are not born with it, do not learn it at school, and, even if they acquire it, are likely to continue to make errors of judgment and method under stress and in the face of conflicting and unpredictable pressures.

Why the Manager Does Not Get the Expected Supervisory Performance

When circumstances change, what the boss said earlier may no longer apply. The boss may have been purposely vague as to what was expected from the manager in order to motivate the manager to work longer hours at greater intensity. The boss may not reward the manager adequately because the manager's bargaining power is weak and the boss has a fixed amount of money or status to dispense.

The boss's primary concern may be protecting his or her own job rather than organizational growth and system maintenance. Therefore, the boss may wish to keep the manager on a tight leash and to focus the manager's energies on satisfying the boss's need for aggrandizement and survival rather than on providing support services to physicians and nurses or acting as patients' advocate. The boss may not want to tell a manager that he or she is doing well, for fear that the manager will slack off or become overconfident. The boss may not want to tell a manager that he or she is doing poorly in certain areas because the boss may think the manager cannot handle criticism. The boss may not want the manager to withdraw whatever contributions he or she is making until the boss can dispense suddenly with the manager's services.

The boss may not explain how what the manager does fits into the larger picture because the boss wants to limit the manager's power by denying the manager information. Or the boss may keep the manager in the dark because he or she does not want to restrain the manager from pursuing a certain course that is opposed by other organizational interests; the manager can thereby deflect antagonism away from the boss and toward himself or herself. Filling the manager in takes time, and the boss may lack adequate time or may accord the manager's needs lower priority than other demands on the boss's time.

The boss may not recognize adequately the manager's contribution or adequately consider the manager as an individual because the boss places a different value on the manager's contribution relative to others than the manager does. It could be that the boss did not choose the manager, does not like him or her, thinks the manager should be working harder or more effectively, or thinks the manager lacks sufficient personal loyalty to the boss or to the organization. The boss may not protect the manager when he or she is wrong because the boss wants to get rid of the manager.

So Where Is Justice?

In short, there are good reasons for you and your boss (and for you and your subordinates) to discuss, define, and attempt to agree upon what performance is required. There are good reasons for each side to explain to the other why agreed-upon performance expectations can or cannot be met.

There are also good reasons why such discussions do not happen more frequently and with better results than they do. You cannot expect justice in organizational life. If you seek the ideal, you may be denied the acceptable. If, however, you are making significant contributions to your organization, if you can demonstrate that you are, and if you are perceived by important persons in the organization as making such contributions, then it is likely that you will be asked to continue to make such contributions, if not in your organization, in some other one. If your expectations are too high relative to the boss's, your expectations are likely to be lowered over time as you become aware of others' perceptions of your contribution, or perhaps you can raise your level of performance. If your expectations are too low relative to the boss's, perhaps you are being taken advantage of or will be unexpectedly rewarded.

VII
Managing Your Team

The essential strategy of leadership in mobilizing power is to recognize the arrays of motives and goals in potential followers, to appeal to those motives by words and action, and to strengthen those motives and goals in order to increase the power of leadership, thereby changing the environment within which both followers and leaders act.

James McGregor Burns

Executives seeking to advance their departments, to answer the claims of competing subordinates, to "protect" their departments against the "aggressions" of other departments as all compete to maintain low operating costs, set production records, prevent accidents—and escape responsibility for them—get credit for ideas contributed and service given, and "to get along and keep out of trouble" with each other and with production workers . . .

Melville Dalton

This chapter deals with who the members of the management team are, working on a new team, recruiting, promoting, and keeping motivated team members, reorganizing the team, working with temporary allies, and managing one's family as members of one's team.

As managers, you face conflicting pressures. On the one hand, you want to reveal yourself and to be loved for who you are. On the other hand, you may wish to merge your managerial and private selves. You may view your private nature as much more important than, and necessarily separate from, your managerial roles, which are lesser and transitory aspects of yourself. You may learn over time how to effectively separate your managerial roles from your private self or how to combine the two in ways that best fit your circumstances.

The manager confronts similar conflicting pressures in dealing with team members. Should you treat your subordinates primarily as important cogs in the organizational machine, or should you respond to them first as persons and only secondarily as workers, or "cogs"? Should your first loyalty be to the person or to the organization, and do you have to choose?

As with many value questions, there is no right or wrong answer. You may be able to generalize your actions and attitudes toward others and yet consistently make appropriate exceptions to any generalizations. Such behavior may be instinctive. In the face of conflicting values you may not be willing to consciously plan your behavior. Our reasons for doing things are often rationalizations after the fact rather than logical and sequential weighings of pros and cons beforehand.

EXAMPLE:

You hire Claire Rogers, fire Victor Alan, and promote Sam Robinson not as a scientific exercise in personnel recruitment, but because you feel that Rogers can do the job, Alan has been given a fair chance, and Robinson has earned his promotion. Your actions are a signal to other managers that they, too, can be rewarded for effective contributions to the organization. You can deny Rogers the data system she needs even though you see the logic of her cause. Firing Alan does not mean that you dislike him or that you will not try to assist him in obtaining a job somewhere else. Promoting Robinson does not mean that you like him.

If you try to do everything yourself, you limit your potential to accomplish goals through others. The nondelegator is unlikely to satisfy the aspirations and expectations of his or her highly educated and aspiring employees. A leader must know when to act, be able to see which goals involve the wants and needs of his or her followers, and be capable of acting in the face of a rapidly changing and often ambiguous environment.

The Inner Core

Two important and very valuable members of your team are your secretary and your administrative assistant—that is, if you are fortunate enough to have them. You may share the services of these individuals with others. Top managers may have more than one secretary or administrative assistant.

Secretaries and administrative assistants will have their own goals and aspirations. Your secretary may be going to school part-time, and your administrative assistant, in a small organization, may function principally as a department head for purchasing and personnel. Some of the tasks your secretary does can be done equally well by a typist, a receptionist, or a clerk. Similarly, some of your administrative assistant's work can be done by a secretary (many secretaries have the title of administrative assistant) or by department heads.

Your Secretary

What you expect from your secretary will depend on mutual preferences, styles, qualifications, experience, and the demands placed on you. Some managers and secretaries function as workaholics together, even travelling frequently to other cities. Others function as interdependent cogs in a larger machine, each of whom has his or her own work to do. Some managers expect their secretaries to respond to patient inquiries and complaints, to correct grammar and spelling, and to write routine letters. Others view the secretary's job as typing, filing, reception, and scheduling, with little use of independent judgment.

Obviously, both you and your secretary should have similar views of what is expected. Whatever your mutual expectations, however, your secretary is perceived by others as an extension of yourself and as your representative. As a manager, you are often unavailable to persons seeking to contact you. If your secretary is brusque, usually pleads ignorance, or is passive and only carries out instructions, people may view your office, rightly or wrongly, as incompetent, unfriendly and poorly managed.

What I have expected from my secretaries is good attendance, pleasantness with me and with persons seeking to contact me, independent thinking so I can avoid mistakes, confidentiality with regard to managerial work, and the ability to solve remediable problems on the spot using their own judgment. I want to be told in advance if some tasks cannot be completed on schedule. I would hope that my secretaries would do urgent work after hours, as long as this is not routinely demanded and they do not have conflicting commitments.

What my secretaries can expect from me is an understanding that I am dependent upon them, rather than that they are dependent upon me. I will explain what I expect and how I think business should be conducted. I will express my appreciation of work that meets higher than acceptable standards. I will advocate the highest possible pay for my secretaries as long as it can be justified relative to the work they perform. I will grant time off if requested, because they have worked extra hours when urgent work had to be completed. I will be considerate of personal needs and yet hold high expectations regarding hours worked, pages typed, or time spent on the job actually working.

An effective secretary can greatly improve your contribution as a manager. Secretaries have another set of managerial ears, which can be invaluable to your understanding of organizational politics. They can advocate for patients or patients' relatives in obtaining remedial action from a department head. They can protect your time by shielding you from persons to whom they or others can respond satisfactorily. Your secretary can make certain that you are available to persons whom you need to see and to whom, for political reasons, you wish to have ready access. Secretaries also manage the files and can, it is hoped, locate quickly what you are searching for, even if the file or paper is in your desk drawer or you have taken it home. Most important, they can respond to others with courtesy and interest. Their response indicates whether you are caring and attentive to visitors' aspirations and expectations.

Your Administrative Assistant

What I have expected from my administrative assistants, administrative residents, or new assistant administrators has been long hours and hard work, a knack for details and accuracy in reporting, a gift for avoiding political controversy, and the ability to listen and to be perceived by others as listening to what they are saying. I have favored persons who get their major gratification from their work rather than from leisure activities and who, after orientation, are able to perform most managerial tasks such as evaluating regulations or analyzing budgets by themselves or with occasional help from others.

What they can expect from me includes telling them what is expected, telling them what my underlying assumptions are in making and implementing important decisions, and assistance with their career planning. They can expect me to set a standard for quality and quantity of their contribution. I will evaluate their performance and suggest ways of improving it. I will show them consideration and respect as individuals.

An effective administrative assistant can greatly augment efficient management by freeing you to deal with more of the demands and claims made upon your time by other persons. (Of course, some managers do not want to do this.) You can accomplish tasks otherwise not feasible, such as a study in depth of the operations of a particular department or program, or an evaluation of new programs or equipment in other organizations. An administrative assistant can spend more time than you could with dissatisfied groups with little power in order to convince them that top management is concerned about their problems, to explain to them why certain solutions are not feasible, and to correct those problems that are remediable.

Peers and Subordinates

Other team members can be divided into line and staff. Line managers include general managers and heads of departments that provide medical care and related support services to physicians and nurses. The radiology department and the laboratory department are examples. Staff managers are those whose departments provide support services to general managers and department heads. Such staff services include finance, marketing, planning, personnel, information services, and public relations.

Because of the nature of their work, line department heads may view themselves primarily as clinicians (or technicians) rather than as managers and may share the goals and viewpoints of the clinical staff. This is particularly true if department heads were promoted to their positions from within and were formerly technicians. The manager should be wary of making demands that conflict with these department heads' loyalty to clinicians.

Staff department heads may function independently because they may possess knowledge that you lack or have access to resources or legitimacy that you do not. They are much less likely, however, to adopt the goals and viewpoints of clinicians, relative to those of general managers.

Expect to both agree and disagree with the same individual on your team depending on the issue. Hospital administrator Victor Alan can deny the demands of Bill Jones, department head in inhalation therapy, for increased departmental salaries, yet attempt to provide the department with additional space to meet its growing needs.

It may be difficult to gain and keep the respect of some department heads and managers. You can seldom escape complaints from, or feelings of favoritism among, department heads relative to their peers, regardless of your attempts to be equitable. Department heads' belief that they receive due process relative to each other can be important in moderating the pain of perceived inequities.

In developing your managerial team, foster a spirit of teamwork. Although team members may be expected to differ from each other on certain issues because of their different constituencies, they should be able to work together after decisions have been reached. You share many of the same expectations and aspirations. You are members of the same organization and have common interests. Can you remain trusting of each other despite occasionally conflicting interests? Not always or completely, but a climate of trust is something valuable and well worth working hard to develop and maintain. When trust permeates an organization, greater attention can be paid to job accomplishment and the obtaining of additional resources. There is less bickering and withdrawal of energy and effort from the job. The importance of developing a climate of trust among managerial team members may explain, in part, the commitment of certain large corporations to promoting from within, assuring lifetime careers for managers, and developing a sense of "family" among managers and workers.

Working on a New Team

Your employment will affect everyone who works with you, particularly anyone who thinks that he or she should have gotten your job. In addition, other workers may feel that your remuneration is out of line with theirs. Be aware of these feelings on the part of others.

It is always difficult to start a new job, especially if requirements of the new job differ significantly from those of your last job or if this is your first job. Your boss should, if possible, make an extra effort during your first few months on the job to make you feel at home and to help you overcome the different and often severe problems of adjusting to a new work environment. Such problems may be compounded if you and your family have made a geographical move as well.

When you start your new job, somebody else's managerial team is already in place. Existing department heads and administrative staff will worry and be uncertain. Some may think that they will benefit from your joining the organization; others may not. You may have been recruited to implement policies that are at variance with those of your predecessor. Your priorities will fit better with the skills, experience, and beliefs of some managers and department heads than with those of others.

As a new manager, you may enter a politically uncertain job environment. But new managers at any level must consider trusting those upon whom they depend. You are more likely to trust people with whom you have worked before than those whom you are meeting for the first time in the new job. You will most likely trust those persons whom you have recruited more than those whom your predecessor recruited, and you are likely to trust persons who recruited you more than persons who did not participate in recruiting you.

When a new manager takes over as chief executive for an entire organization, the wonder is not that so many department heads and administrative staff resign or are fired, but that so many choose or are chosen to stay on. The reasons for this are varied and relate in part to the job options and past job satisfaction of incumbents. There are also only so many things that the new top manager can do at any one time, and effective recruitment of managerial personnel is often a lengthy and difficult process. The new top manager may see most department heads and administrative staff as technically proficient and politically harmless. The incumbents may be eager to demonstrate their loyalty to their new boss, or they may hold back.

It is not easy to readjust your thinking and performance for a new top manager. This is especially true when the new chief executive's personality and view of the job contrast sharply with those of your previous boss. It is difficult to respond to the push of new managers who may not remain long and to the pull of old managers who may be on their way out. This is not a time for pursuing new managerial initiatives. Rather, you should concentrate on support activities—and there is usually more demand for this kind of managerial contribution than you can effectively supply anyway.

Recruiting and Promoting

Many health services organizations do a poor job of recruiting. They do not devote sufficient resources to the effort, and it is not organized well enough. Nor is the recruitment effort subject to sufficient planning and evaluation. Contrast the effort that goes into selecting a $300,000 piece of equipment with a useful life of 12 years to the effort that goes into selecting a nurse aide who makes $12,000 a year and who may work for the organization for 30 years.

Effective recruitment of a managerial team (and of all employees) can enhance the reputation of a health services organization. There may be political repercussions when certain job applicants are rejected. Every job applicant is a potential patient or relative of somebody important. Often your organization will not be able to recruit its first choice among candidates because of money, location, another job offer, or for other reasons. Thus it is important to show courtesy to all candidates. Recruiters should respond promptly to all candidates and tell them whether they are being seriously considered, what the nature of the recruiting process is, and when they can expect to learn the outcome.

There are benefits and costs in promoting technicians to managerial posts. The skills, experience, and beliefs necessary to excel at being a technical staff member or department head are often not the same as those required to excel as a manager. Doing a job well is different from motivating others to do a job well. Once a promotion is given to a loyal, hardworking subordinate, it is difficult to demote him or her. If a technician is promoted to department head and then does not work out from the manager's point of view, the organization may have lost a good technician as well as not having found a good department head (and having lowered departmental or unit morale).

Knowing the organization well is both an advantage and a disadvantage for new managers. They may accept current structure and function. Others in the organization may persist in viewing them in terms of their past positions and responsibilities. The organization may not expect as much from an inside appointee as it would from someone new. Newly promoted managers may be vulnerable if they lack the formal qualifications usually required for such positions, such as a master's degree in health services management. Further their judgment may be open to question if, lacking such formal qualifications, they make some otherwise understandable mistakes and errors soon after they are appointed.

Keeping Your Team Motivated

There are no simple ways of keeping your team motivated or, for that matter, of keeping yourself motivated. The aphorism, "If it ain't broken, don't fix it," also applies to human beings and to organizational design or process. If individuals are performing well, don't interfere with them.

Some persons do not need to be motivated by anyone else. These self-starters will, if adequately informed and supported, work with energy and grace to accomplish mutually agreed-upon goals. In addition, they may make helpful suggestions for changes in response to changing circumstances, and may give you needed feedback on aspects of your own performance.

On the other hand, there are persons who will not or cannot change their performance. If the organization is large enough, there may be other positions in which such persons can perform adequately. If not, you have to fire them, never a pleasant process. An organization is not a democracy. It exists for limited purposes rather than as an end in itself. If ineffective persons are permitted to draw paychecks, their work must be done by others, be done ineffectively, or not be done at all. Presumably, in the last analysis the patient or the client suffers.

You must focus your energies on motivating those persons who, with help, will be able to perform effectively. People can be put (justly or unjustly) into categories such as "works well without help," "works well with help," and "cannot work sufficiently well, even with help." The same persons may fall into different categories at different times or in regard to different aspects of their work. Categorizing accurately may be difficult, as excellent subordinates and staff can make ineffective managers or department heads look good for a while, and effective managers or department heads may be temporarily incapacitated by a death in the family, illness, or other personal reasons.

When you are dissatisfied with a team member's performance, you must ask yourself why. Are you dissatisfied with the results of the performance or with the style? Put another way, is this a matter of the team member's lack of knowledge, poor judgment, or bad attitudes? Has the person always performed poorly? If not, why is the person performing poorly now?

It is important to ask the manager or department head why his or her performance has been below your expectations. You should do this privately and confidentially and perhaps also not in your office, which may be viewed as a threatening environment. Once you suspect that one of your team members is performing under par it makes sense to document the circumstances. This should not be a substitute for the regular formal evaluation process.

As a manager, you must ask yourself whether you are part of a team member's problem. Have you made clear what kind and level of performance you expect? Did the team member agree to this standard? If you do not trust the manager or department head, what facts can be marshalled to support your judgment? You should ask the team member if there is any way you can be more helpful to him or her.

Expect people to respond differently to your criticism. Some will agree with you on the facts, deny any generalizatons, explain what went wrong, and promise to do better. Others will disagree on the facts or on their interpretation. Some will disagree on what a definition of acceptable performance is. Others will claim that outward events over which they had no control interfered with their performance.

After you and the team member have discussed the problem, the team member can come to one of several conclusions. He or she can accept the criticism constructively and attempt to change what behavior he or she can. Generally speaking, it is easier for a person to stop or to start doing something than it is to change the way he or she does something. The more specific a goal is, the easier it is to know whether the team member can meet it. There is little a team member can do when accused of having a bad attitude; it is easier to initiate fewer conversations with physicians than to change the tone of those conversations.

It is important that you try to communicate to the team member that your criticism is not meant personally; rather, you are attempting to be helpful so that he or she can meet the goals that both of you have set. The team member must first genuinely perceive that there is a problem. He or she should recognize that if you as the manager perceive there is a problem then a problem exists, even if the team member is blameless. In disclosing your concerns, you run the risk that, rather than changing his or her behavior, the team member will withdraw and cover himself or herself, steadily arguing for lower managerial expectations and blaming outside influences if such expectations are not met.

It is at this point that you must act to get rid of the team member. If you lack specific documentation, the alerted team member may be careful not to give you any specific reasons to fire him or her. Reasons can always be manufactured, but the situation will have become decidedly unpleasant. Sometimes this is unavoidable, if only because you wish to give each member of the team a fair chance.

A more useful approach may be to accept the fact that, even if a team member has certain abilities, the two of you have conflicting personalities. You may have different beliefs about organizational policy or style. This is a problem for both of you, one that you should discuss (calmly, it is hoped), to see what can be done. If there is a serious conflict, you and the team member have several choices. Either or both of you can resign. You can deny the problem, insist that each can meet mutual expectations, and attempt to do so. You can work to undermine each other. In this situation, managers usually tell the team member that, if he or she does not wish to resign, the manager will fire him or her. You must be able to trust team members upon whom you and the organization rely, and you cannot trust anyone after you have told him or her that there are basic personality conflicts between you or that you have major differences regarding organizational priorities or ways of conducting business.

The whole process may seem decidedly unfair from the point of view of the team member, department head, or administrative staff member, but injustice is a management reality. Managers are paid and esteemed for being able to deal effectively with risk and uncertainty. There is no shortage of candidates for managerial positions, and top managers themselves can be asked to resign or be fired. Managers must be humane, remembering that "There but for the grace of God go I."

Sometimes, being asked to resign, or even being fired, is the best thing that can happen to someone. The position might never have worked out. A new job opportunity may be a promotion. Even if the new job pays less, working conditions may be better and the team member may feel more secure. The team member may be relieved at no longer having to attempt a job or to get along with a manager when neither was really feasible, given the manager's and the team member's differing skills, beliefs, and experience. Team members may learn what their strengths and weaknesses really are, how others perceive them, who their friends are, and what it is they really want to do. They may strengthen ties with family or friends.

Team members may have learned how to avoid an avoidable termination, and this knowledge may enable them to do the same type of work better somewhere else. Of course, some people never learn. And some people are never given a second chance.

Reorganizing Your Team

A new manager is given three envelopes by his or her predecessor and is instructed to open one each time he or she encounters difficulties on the job. Things are not going well, and the new manager opens the first envelope. The message inside reads, "Blame things on your predecessor." As working conditions worsen, the manager opens the second envelope. The message inside reads, "Now is the time to reorganize." As things keep on getting worse, the manager opens the third envelope. The message reads, "Prepare three envelopes."

Reorganizing managerial responsibilities will probably not solve the most important problems you face, but it can shield you from certain problems until perhaps you understand the causes of them better. You can gain needed time to respond more effectively to problems.

Reorganizing is not always a cover-up for not having done things right in the first place. Circumstances change. New people join the organization, and team members who have been around for a while leave. When a member of the managerial team leaves, for whatever reason, it is a good time to reassess the vacated position. Ask whether the tasks and responsibilities that go with the job can be handled more effectively by someone else in the organization. Decide whether you or another manager should take over certain functions of the existing position, perhaps giving up some of your own functions.

When a manager leaves, his or her position may stay vacant for a while, if only because he or she left suddenly and it has taken a while to fill the position appropriately. Leaving a position vacant for several months may be desirable in order to find out more about the former occupant's contribution and any future occupant's potential contribution to organizational effectiveness. The effects of a manager's leaving may not be noticeable until considerable time has elapsed, however.

There are benefits and costs in reorganizing managerial responsibilities regularly, even if the management team remains the same. A benefit is that each manager develops a clearer understanding of the total organization and of the problems faced by other managers in other parts of the organization. The organization becomes less dependent on specific managers because expertise is shared. Effective decision making may be facilitated because managers' judgment may become more balanced and they will share a base of information. Evaluation of managers is facilitated because a different manager may be the only significant variable affecting unit performance. Large organizations are able to rotate managers more frequently and to give them greater career mobility within the organization. This enhances stability and breadth of managerial response throughout the organization.

On the other hand, while some managers like and can respond effectively to certain challenges, others do not like challenges or certain ones and cannot respond well to them. If you are performing effectively, given your present responsibilities, why make a switch and begin doing something you do not really want to know how to do? You may have spent years learning how to handle your present responsibilities effectively; you may have earned the trust of your peers, and elicited outstanding performance from a number of highly trained subordinates. Now you are likely to be ineffective while you are learning your new duties. Some managers work better with certain responsibilities and with certain subordinates than with others.

Small organizations have an advantage over large organizations in that their managers tend to be less specialized; however, each manager's contribution may be relatively more important to adequate organizational performance. When a manager leaves or is incapacitated, therefore, it tends to be a larger crisis for small organizations than for large organizations.

EXAMPLE:

Bob Bellows is director of the department of management information systems for Urban HMO, which has 800,000 enrollees. Bellows reports to Clark Weiss, the vice-president for hospitals and health centers. Wyatt Burns, the vice-president for planning and support services, argues that Urban's management information systems department is many years behind current technology. Burns says his people are not getting the information they need, that Weiss does not understand the problem and has ignored Burns' requests for overhauling management information systems.

In response to Burns' complaints, Walter Ormes, the HMO president, has to take the following factors into consideration. He believes that Burns will do a more competent job than Weiss in directing the management information systems department, but Burns is likely to fire Bellows, the present department head, who has worked loyally for the organization for 11 years (Burns has been with Urban for twenty years). Bellows, however, has not been able to keep up with technological developments. Burns' changes will cost a lot of money and result in a lot of temporary disruptions. Weiss will regard the shifting of responsibility as a slap in the face. Ormes is not convinced that the ineffectiveness of management information systems is as serious as Burns says for HMO performance requirements now. But Ormes admits that the system may well have to be upgraded significantly in the next three to five years.

Reorganizing has important symbolic as well as substantive aspects for Ormes, Weiss, and Burns. It tells managers and subordinates which areas, units, or managers are considered problems and are losing power, and which are meeting managerial expectations and gaining power. If organizational responsibility for management information systems is shifted from Weiss to Burns, and if Burns can demonstrate improved performance and contribution to organizational effectiveness in the next two years, Burns will gain power relative to Weiss.

If, on the other hand, service deteriorates significantly after the change and after Burns has fired Bellows, or if Burns cannot demonstrate the department's enhanced contribution to organizational decision making, Weiss will gain power relative to Burns. If HMO premiums have to be raised because of increases in information systems costs and because of decreases in the number of new enrollees, Ormes may downgrade Burns, even if the shift in managerial responsibilities has little to do with increased costs per member month. Burns might be extremely successful in reorganizing management information systems, leave the HMO, and found his own consulting firm. Does this leave Ormes and Urban HMO better or worse off?

Working with Temporary Allies

Most large health services organizations consist of many organizational participants, each with only partial authority over the other, who work with and against each other in shifting coalitions. Such coalitions create temporary allies. For hospital managers, temporary allies can include trustees, physicians, department heads, community officials, regulators, and other managers in his or her own or other organizations.

Managers work together with temporary allies when their interests coincide. They work against each other when their interests conflict. They should be able to retain each other's trust and respect under changing circumstances by paying attention to each other as individuals, opposing each other without violating certain behavioral rules, and committing themselves to what often becomes a slow, tedious, and ineffective process of decision making because of the need to pay sufficient attention to due process for all parties.

Issues on which you and your temporary allies disagree can be categorized from your perspective as: important and susceptible to compromise, important and not susceptible to compromise, or unimportant. You can certainly give in on or do nothing about issues in the last two categories. You can attempt to gain additional allies or influence present allies through persuasion or inducement based on your authority as an expert; or you can try to shift their attention or alter their perceptions. You can do all of the above, but you will destroy trust and respect by publicly agreeing with opponents and privately working against them.

What you have going for you in working with temporary allies is your organizational legitimacy as a manager—you are supposed to act in such a way as to meet your responsibilities to your department or the entire organization. Managers are usually supposed to be coordinating organizational activities and persons. You should have the time, information, and focus necessary to build effective coalitions. Your position as organizational spokesman and coordinator is subject to challenge, however, by those who may have the power to remove you or to curb your power. They may perceive you as being merely an additional participant or interest group within the organization and as an ineffective manager. They may see you as being paid not to make problems (if that is how they view your attempts to enhance organizational effectiveness), but to avoid or alleviate problems (that is, to provide support and get out of the way).

When you are facing ambiguities about what your responsibilities really are and are uncertain about what would result from either action or inaction on your part, you must pay careful attention to communication, especially with temporary allies. In working with temporary allies, you are trying to communicate with people who may not trust you. They know that your interests and theirs conflict, at least on some issues, hence they constantly seek clues as to where you really stand, what you really think, and how you really feel about them. Many such allies have primary interests outside your organization, such as taking care of patients, running businesses, or regulating other organizations. This means that many issues which are important to you will be unimportant to them and vice versa. Therefore, you may be able to accomplish a great deal, so long as you do not interfere with what they think is important.

When policy interests differ and you are meeting your organizational responsibilities as you and your supervisors have defined them, it may be easier for those who oppose your policy to avoid the issues and attempt to discredit you personally. To the extent that others view you as not to be trusted, they will certainly oppose your policy. If you are not trusted, you will have to spend an extraordinary amount of time documenting and communicating what your policy is and why others have no reason to fear it. I want to emphasize here that, given the power structure of most health services organizations, you cannot allow yourself to be mistrusted. If you cannot convince temporary allies to see things your way, you must at least persuade them that you are honest and predictable and that you understand their concerns. You cannot achieve this unless you spend time with them, listen to them, and demonstrate by your behavior that their concerns matter to you.

Managing Your Family

EXAMPLE:
Dwight Robbins, the administrator of the Henry Poor Neighborhood Health Center (NHC), is highly esteemed for his managerial contribution by Cal Calderone, the chief executive officer of Highsmith Hospital. This is why Calderone promoted Robbins from assistant hospital administrator to administrator of the NHC. Nevertheless, Calderone has become aware that Robbins is absent from work frequently now that his wife, Marlene, has become a full-time doctoral student. Robbins now has child care responsibilities that take up a lot of his time. When Calderone discusses this with Robbins, Robbins responds that he carries out the responsibilities of his job, that he must be absent on occasion, and that he will continue to be absent because one of his children is chronically ill and his wife cannot stay home on certain days of the week.

Contrast Robbins with Claire Rogers, director of nursing at Highsmith Hospital. Her husband, Henry, is a tremendous asset in Rogers' work. He supports her and is knowledgeable about her job. Henry is a gracious host and spends a considerable amount of time with the spouses of nurses, especially the spouses of nurses who have started working recently at Highsmith Hospital. Henry is active in local politics and has made several local connections that are useful to his wife.

Your spouse, children, parents, siblings, friends, lovers, and ex-spouses may be seen as members of your managerial team because they affect how others view you, how you function, and how you feel about yourself. Your spouse and children can provide you with support, respect, and love. Child care responsibilities can complicate and dilute performance at work. Your spouse or parents may have negative feelings about your work or the persons with whom you work. When both spouses work, there may be substantial conflict between their career ambitions and emotional needs.

Busy managers often find it difficult to devote sufficient time to family members. It is one thing not to be married, or to be married and not have children, and to work 70 hours a week, 50 weeks a year for several years. It is another to do so when your spouse works, you have three preschool children, and you have made a geographic change recently because of an important promotion.

Family can be a tremendous assistance in launching and fostering managerial careers. If your career is in a small town and your family is well known and regarded, other people will be likely to trust you because they feel that you will probably take their values into account when you are making and implementing important decisions. Social relationships can significantly affect your chances as a manager. While jealousies and antagonisms among workers' spouses are notorious for adversely affecting work relationships, cooperative and supportive relationships can work just as effectively in the opposite direction. Friends made through volunteer work can also help. You earn trust by helping others when there is nothing obviously "in it" for you. By helping others attain goals that are important to them, you may find it easier to induce them to help your organization or to dilute potential negative reactions toward it.

Interaction with persons in the community is a useful way of getting feedback about how your organization is perceived by those who use and do not use its services. Persons who are not directly involved in the politics of your organization may be more objective about the quality and availability of its services or why certain groups of persons use or do not use your facility or program.

Managing health services organizations is probably a poor career choice for people who cherish privacy. This is not to say that you cannot be successful at work and lead a separate, private life away from the job. However, managers work longer hours than most other persons, and they are likely to have more work-related responsibilities to carry out after hours. Away from work, especially in smaller communities, people will tend to view you first as the local health services manager and second as a private person. For those of you who like socializing, your position as health services manager can obviously be advantageous. Officials of other organizations will tend to respect your position and look to you for participation in civic and charitable affairs.

For most of you, work is no substitute for loving relationships—and such relationships usually cannot endure without your devoting adequate time and energy to them. Some managers may not be capable of loving relationships or may find them less important. For others, such relationships may develop and endure even if very little time is spent on them. My guess is that too many managers spend too little time with their loved ones and that they suffer worse relationships because of it. Given all the extra hours that managers work, I believe more managers should take some time off during regular working hours. Also, they should consider taking their vacations with those they love in places far away from work. Some managers enjoy taking their spouses to work-related meetings or conventions; for others, it means either devoting inadequate attention to the work at hand or to the spouse.

Most of you require private time, periods of complete rest, in order to revive yourself and to think deeply and well about your work. In what directions do you want to devote more or less effort? How can your goals and the organization's goals be better accomplished? What do you want to accomplish in your working life? Such thinking time can be gained by blocking out half days, full days, or weeks on your calendar or by taking long walks or driving long hours before or after work. In any case, thinking time is valuable, and you should build some of it into your schedule.

VIII
Working With Physicians

With just a slight difference in emphasis, or even a different way of lighting Redford, a movie could have been made about a strong yet self-righteous man who didn't know how to gain allies or when to fight and when to bargain, and so lost when he held the cards to win.

Pauline Kael

The basic struggle is initially between the administrator and the medical staff. They are in constant contact, and their interests are often so divergent that conflict rather than cooperation is the rule.

Roman Yanda

All organizations are in a sense political jungles, some more so than others, with a limited supply of money, power, and status in relation to the claims made on these resources. Under such circumstances, how can a manager work with physicians to make an effective contribution? Such a relationship is called "conditional cooperation" by Hugh Heclo and "conflictive equilibrium" by Richard Saltman and David Young.

The manager has to understand what physicians believe he or she should be doing, how to influence physicians, working together, investing and spending the manager's scarce political capital, and how to cope with physician-dominated committees. These are the sections of this chapter. The perspectives of both manager and physician are presented, and avenues for mutual accommodation are explored.

Rules of the Game

Critical to working with physicians is finding out what they think you ought to be doing. What they think may differ from what you were told in graduate school that health service managers are supposed to do. It may also differ from what your boss thinks you should be doing.

Richard Cyert and James March view the organization as a coalition of individuals. As a manager, you focus on the participants in your particular "region"—either temporal or functional. After a brief period, you can identify the most important members of the coalition. You should be able to specify fairly quickly who will attempt to oppose or delay the making and implementing of managerial decisions, at least in your region.

As a manager (and presumably interested in job security unless you are young or wealthy) your objectives are to stay out of others' regions, protect your own region, make sure you know what minimum adequate performance is in your own region, and perform to meet at least that minimum.

Physicians also have their regions. A common mistake of new managers is violating physicians' regions. You may assume that you can help "straighten things out" or improve patient care, but, to physicians, things may be working out just as they should be. Physicians may dislike the way you are trying to help, or they may define their problems differently from you. You may have similar difficulties in managing your own region, and physicians will urge you to attend to those difficulties first. You may be under the mistaken impression that some part of a physician's region is yours. Such mistakes are tolerated for the first few months of your tenure; however, if you persist in them, physicians will take what they see as appropriate action.

A second mistake of new managers is allowing physicians to violate their regions. As a manager, you can lose your job if you are perceived as not contributing sufficiently to organizational effectiveness.

Responding to Complainants

If physicians are dissatisfied with performance in your region, you should try to learn the specifics of the complaint, find out if the facts are accurate, learn the causes of the problem (if there is a problem), and then carefully plan what you intend to do about the complaint and the complainant, how, and when.

You should communicate your findings to the complainant. It is desirable to have remedied whatever problem there was before you even get back to the complainant officially. It is essential in dealing with a complainant to show that you are listening, to show empathy for the complainant's feelings, and to show concern. When you report back to a complainant, you should be able to explain what parts of the problem you can or cannot solve, and when. If you cannot solve the problem, tell the complainant why.

Consider Item 16, in Chapter 11, in which Benjamin Ringo, the chief of pediatrics at Glory Hospital complains to administrator Victor Alan about staffing in the intensive care nursery. Alan attaches the incident report sent to him by Lydia Bailey, director of nursing. He explains what happened and why. He also explains why, although he does not wish it, the situation may recur. Bailey discusses the pros and cons of closing the unit, which Alan opposes as not being in the best interests of the community. Side issue: Ringo is trying to get Alan to fire Bailey because she is not making the contribution to quality of care that he thinks a nursing director should be making at Glory Hospital.

There are several explanations for why a physician complains and why you, as a manager, do not find the complaint to be valid. The physician may be mistaken as to the seriousness or frequency of a problem. He or she may be correct about the problem but lack evidence to validate the complaint. You may believe that the physician is distorting reality to gain other ends. The physician may wish to keep you from making claims upon him or her, or the physician may be trying to get, fairly or unfairly, better service from you.

In validating a complaint, you should search out other physicians who may have a problem similar to the complainant's. Even if, after investigation, you are satisfied that the complaint is not sufficiently valid to take "remedial" action, you may have a problem if the complainant is politically powerful and persistent. As a manager, you then have several alternatives, none of them desirable. You can delay and hope that either the complainant or the problem will go away. You can attempt to gain allies to combat the complainant's position on a particular issue. You can agree with the complainant and delay implementation. You can follow the complainant's wishes, even if the complaint is not valid, thereby possibly antagonizing someone else who is less powerful and running the risk of encouraging other invalid complaints.

You should attempt to determine whether complainants are merely trying to squeeze out every drop of advantage in terms of improved service or whether they are trying to affect you personally. In the latter case, you should respond to the complainant only officially. You must develop a file to protect yourself should the complainant insist that you be called to account for your response or lack of one. Such calling to account may be unlikely, because you can still be useful to the complainant and to others on this or other matters. If the complainant goes to your superior, you must be able to defend yourself in regard to both substance and process. If you are justified, do not worry—unless there are other reasons your superior wants to get rid of you. If so, your superior can always terminate your services without validating physician complaints merely by informing you of "personality conflicts" between you and important physicians.

To look at matters more positively, what happens when you are dealing with a powerful complainant to whom you are not directly accountable can indicate to some extent the strength of your own position. A proportion of such complainants are not as powerful as they or you think they are. Their complaints may be discounted by other powerful physicians or trustees because they are known to complain regularly and to have unrealistic expectations, even when their complaints are valid. As to the remainder of invalid complaints by physicians, you must depend upon your ability to analyze the complaint and document its invalidity or the reasons why it cannot be resolved as the complainant wishes. Or you can refer the complaint to the next higher level of authority. You can then defend yourself, if it comes to that, in terms of your record on other issues, your responses to other complaints and complainants, or your documented contributions to organizational effectiveness and your earned trust in having adequately met the expectations of key physicians and others.

A proportion of the complaints from physicians are valid, and acting upon them promptly makes sense, even if you have other problems of equal or even greater priority. To do otherwise could endanger the contributions the physician is making to the organization.

The Physician Perspective

In working with physicians, it is useful for you to understand their perspective, the extent to which they have a stake in the organization, and how they view managers. According to Eliot Freidson, physicians have been trained to think of themselves as unique individuals with the exclusive right to practice medicine. The physician's growing dependence on organizations is a major concern of many practitioners.

Freidson has characterized medicine as a consulting, not a scientific or scholarly, profession. Physicians value medical responsibility and clinical expertise rather than abstract knowledge. Their aim is action, not knowledge. As a result, Freidson says, "unnecessary surgery and over-prescribing may be a natural consequence of decision rules rather than of carelessness and ignorance." Patients, too, want physicians to act. Physicians see a biased sample of patients—those for whom whatever they are doing works or who believe it works. Patients who are dissatisfied or who die are not there to confront physicians with failure.

Freidson points out that physicians work in collegial groups built up by patronage and boycott. Such groups are fairly well segregated from each other. This situation does not tend to correct or eliminate poor physician performance. Being supervised, for many physicians, is synonymous with being a student in medical school, which they remember as distinctly unpleasant. Physicians, Freidson continues, have no special expertise in social organization or the management of treatment.

Managers cannot assume that the services physicians provide are of uniform, adequate quality or that they are medically necessary. In a study by David Kessner et al. of 2,150 poor children in Washington, D.C., 70 percent of the children wearing glasses could see as well without them; only one-third of the children whose blood tests showed them to be anemic were formally diagnosed as such and treated for the disorder. Lester Breslow indicates that in 1967, about a year after starting the Medicaid program in California, "hundreds of physicians treating sizeable numbers of Medicaid patients gave on the average of 50 to 100 more injections (other than immunizations) per 100 patient visits." David Rosenhan cites an experiment in which persons gained admission to mental hospitals with feigned symptoms. Once in the hospitals, their malingering was not recognized; when they stopped exhibiting symptoms, hospital staff were incapable of noting the difference.

Franz Ingelfinger has indicated that 90 percent of the visits by patients to doctors are caused by conditions that are either self-limited or beyond the capabilities of medicine. Marcia Millman argues that "although doctors may have differences and rivalry among themselves with regard to defining, blaming, and acting on mistakes, all doctors will join hands and close ranks against patients and the public" (and against the manager, I might add).

Freidson asserts that many questions of medical care are social, not professional, questions, although they are not often addressed as such. Examples include information regarding alternative methods of treatment and the freedom to change treatment, patient convenience versus provider convenience, and decisions concerning institutionalization. For example, consultants may be used to provide legal protection for the physician without even asking the patient's permission.

The point of the above paragraphs is not to belittle or denigrate physicians. Many physicians do work well in organizations, provide care of adequate or superior quality, and cause managers little or no trouble. Perhaps these physicians should be causing managers more trouble, if that would mean assuring better service to patients. Even if much of medical care is not cost-effective, the amelioration physicians do provide is often valued greatly by patients, who continue to regard at least their own physicians highly. What is important for managers to realize is that physicians and managers have legitimately different interests and that physicians are not always right about what they define as medical matters. Managers should enter the "medical" arena with extreme caution, but they must enter it occasionally, for this is where the stakes are often highest for the patient.

Physician Expectations

Physicians expect to be recognized for the important contributions they make to health services organizations and to American society (physician status in the United States is higher than that of health services managers or other professionals). Physicians expect managers to give due, and sometimes undue, consideration to their livelihoods and their egos.

Attending physicians, as Mark Blumberg indicates, earn 50 to 60 percent more per hour for hospital services than for office services. Many physicians are totally dependent upon health services organizations for their remuneration.

Physicians guard their status relative to peers in their organization and in other organizations. They want to determine their own working conditions and will fight vigorously any decision that negatively affects "their" space, "their" equipment, or "their" personnel. Physicians require adequate support services to treat patients.

Physicians do not wish their time to be wasted or to spend more time at organizational meetings than is absolutely necessary. Most of them work 55 to 60 hours a week. Physicians, like everyone else, want to be consulted about policy decisions they feel will affect them, both before policy is made and during its implementation.

Managerial Response

If your employment is dependent in part on not antagonizing physicians, why can you not meet physicians' expectations, many of which seem quite reasonable? To begin with, you do not control the distribution of many of the organizational resources that physicians want and expect. There are limited amounts available. If every physician has similar access to you or to organizational resources, none of them is better off than any other. Some of them wish to be or deserve to be better off than others.

Financial pressures on the organization may cause a deterioration in the physician's working conditions. Paying customers may move out of a hospital's service area. Expenditure ceilings may be placed on the hospital by regulators.

Physicians' interests often conflict with organizational goals or with the interests of other physicians. Trustees may wish to establish ambulatory services for the underserved poor and handicapped, whereas attending physicians oppose the services as potentially competitive with their private practices. Some physicians in a group practice may want their partners to produce more or to make less money; certain of their partners will disagree.

Managers and physicians may have different concepts of wasting time. The time that physicians spend at committee meetings is time away from patient care and time for which they are not being paid, whereas managers are being paid and are doing their jobs properly when they attend meetings. (Your hourly rate of compensation does tend to fall as you attend more and longer meetings after hours.)

Sometimes events move too quickly for you to consult adequately with certain physicians whom you would like to contact. Sometimes physician officials do not spend enough energy and time communicating with staff in their departments or on their committees. Sometimes staff physicians do not attend meetings that are organized for communicating with them or do not thoroughly read letters and memos that are sent to them to keep them informed.

Sometimes physician expectations are not met because they are unrealistic or unfair. Or even when they are realistic and fair, they may not be met because other physicians who are organizational officials have personal difficulties with a physician or have doubts about his or her work or character.

The Managerial Perspective

Given that managerial and physician goals sometimes conflict and that physicians may lack commitment to organizational goals, what kind of behavior do managers expect from physicians with whom they must deal on a regular basis?

Managerial Expectations

You may expect recognition for your position and your person. After all, you can be helpful or obstructive to the interests of specific physicians, if not to all physicians. You may expect personal commitment from physicians to organizational goals, at least to the extent prescribed in organizational bylaws and departmental and medical staff rules and regulations. You may expect physicians to fulfill certain organizational responsibilities, such as attending medical staff meetings or committee meetings of which the physician is chairman. You may expect physicians who disagree with you on policy matters not to take it out on you personally (since your support is necessary to them on other important issues). You may expect physicians not to waste your time. If physicians have a complaint about the food or about cleanliness, you may expect them to complain to the department head or assistant administrator responsible rather than to you as associate administrator or chief executive officer. (On the other hand, you may not want physicians to follow such a chain of command, in order that you may provide more personal service.) You may expect to be consulted on policy decisions made by medical officials when their decisions affect your responsibilities. Such decisions may concern appointment to and composition of medical staff committees in a not-for-profit hospital, or the employment of legal and accounting staff in a large, multispecialty group practice.

Physician Response

Many of these managerial expectations seem reasonable. If physicians are increasingly dependent on the organization in which they work, then why do they not meet such expectations more regularly? To begin with, physicians may not view managers as you view yourself. Physicians may believe that your responsibilities are primarily to support physicians and nurses, who take care of patients, rather than to coordinate activities among clinical and support services and to relate the organization to outside groups and organizations.

Physicians may fear that you will act to curb their powers and so wish to oppose you on the issues, even if this means diluting contributions you could otherwise make to organizational survival and growth. Some physicians fear that you will seek control over their working conditions, incomes, and status. Such fears may be well founded, especially as physicians become more plentiful and as managerial performance becomes more critical to the effectiveness of larger and more complex health services organizations.

Physicians may disagree bitterly with you on policy. They may feel that your "persuading" of other physicians and trustees is unfair. They may believe that you interpret unfairly to board members their principled opposition to managerial initiatives as personal attacks on you and that you communicate your interpretation to board members. In such circumstances, physicians may feel justified in attacking you personally—either to your face or behind your back—to other physicians and trustees. Physicians may have a direct conflict of interest with certain organizational goals. A radiologist on the hospital staff may be in competition with the radiology department. An internist may refer all laboratory work to a competing for-profit laboratory. A salaried psychiatrist may have a private office where he sees patients after hours in competition with the hospital. On the other hand, attending physicians may suffer financially when they devote too much time to hospital business. Their health or family life may suffer if, after accepting additional hospital responsibilities, they do not reduce the number of hours they spend in the office.

Most hospitals lack effective accountability systems for medical officials. For example, a chief of surgery may be elected to serve a one-year term on a rotational basis. Such a chief cannot be expected to hold other surgeons accountable for the quality of their work, their attendance at meetings, and so forth. The chief, in turn, may not be held accountable in any formal way to a higher hospital authority. The same lack of formal accountability may characterize a prepaid group practice, where medical officials are not held accountable to governing bodies or chief operating partners and cannot be or are not removed when they do not meet minimal performance requirements.

Finally, physicians may not meet your managerial expectations because they do not trust you personally, they do not like you, or they do not respect you. This may be because of something you have done or because of something they fear you may do.

Influencing Physicians

Despite the inherent difficulties in influencing physician behavior, there are compelling organizational reasons for trying to. What are the opportunities that you as a manager can grasp and pursue? If physicians trust you, they are more apt to go along with you, but will they trust you if you do not give them everything they want?

You must show good judgment. Worry about making too many decisions. Worry about making decisions too soon or too late. But make decisions. If decisions will affect them, then by all means involve physicians, at appropriate levels, in implementation. Before making a decision, you must have all the relevant facts at your disposal, assuming they can be gotten at an acceptable cost. If not, you must admit to physicians who question your judgment that you do not have but will get the facts or that it does not make sense to try. Your reputation for honesty and trustworthiness is usually more important to physicians than your technical knowledge.

Do not promise too much. It is better that the policy you urge not be adopted than that promised outcomes fail to materialize when you predicted them. Usually, you must retreat after you make a mistake or lose a decision. Sometimes it is not important if you lose; doing so can demonstrate your fallibility or stimulate awareness of an issue and the consequences if a decision is not made now. Later, if you are proven right, your judgment will count more heavily when the next such issue is raised.

You may do favors for physicians. As Robert Strauss, former chairman of the Democratic National Committee, has said, "Doing favors is like money in the bank." However, what you may regard as a favor, the physician may see as only doing your job. When you need their support, physicians may have more costly favors to pay back to other physicians. You may have extended yourself more than anyone else in the organization to help certain physicians, but they are less dependent on the hospital than they are upon the goodwill of other physicians, who refer patients to them.

Charles Lindblom indicates three ways of influencing others: exchange, authority, and persuasion. Physicians will go along with you on an issue in exchange for scarce resources of program commitment, space, budget, or personnel. Physicians will not oppose you if they believe you have the relevant expertise or experience on a certain issue. Physicians will agree with you on policy when you can persuade them that what you want them to do is in their best interest.

Even when you agree with physicians on the issues, you may have to hold them back if there are major risks involved in immediate full-scale implementation of an approved initiative. You can be helpful to physicians by making their claims upon resources more realistic and therefore more obtainable.

Sources of Physician Power

Physicians have several sources of power in dealing with managers. They may have certain legal rights, as stated in the organization's bylaws, medical staff bylaws, or contracts specifying the terms of their employment. Physicians often have substantial informal power because of the allegiance they have earned from nurses and technicians through their skill in taking care of patients or through personal or professional favors. Physicians often have direct access to important board members and community leaders, each of whom, after all, has a personal physician. Physicians may belong to professional organizations that protect their rights as physicians. For example, hospital radiologists are members of the hospital medical staff. They may have their own management contract with the hospital. They may be members of the American Medical Association, the state medical association, and their own specialty association of radiologists.

Saltman and Young emphasize that physicians as a group maintain control over hospital decision-making processes by maximizing the uncertainty that they will perform their functions as expected. Physicians often have the power to admit their patients to other hospitals or to set up competing organizations, at least for the provision of ambulatory services.

A final source of power is the physician's technical knowledge. When the physician defines a situation as a medical emergency, managers jump now and ask questions later.

Sources of Management Power

Managers know a great deal more than most physicians do about finance, regulation, accreditation, corporate planning, fund raising, personnel policy, and other operations in health services organizations. The executive officer of a not-for-profit hospital or an HMO is selected by a governing board and may enjoy special access to board members that many physicians lack. Board members may perceive managers as their delegates, and physicians as individuals whom they wish their delegates to confront. Managers have access to information that is not usually available to or not easily understood by many physicians (in the amount of time they are willing to devote to interpreting such data). Managers are seen by physicians, to varying extents, as adjudicators among physicians when they differ as to allocation of resources. Managers are seen as appropriately adjudicating certain claims on limited organizational resources by physicians and nonphysicians.

Managers may have certain responsibilities because of their employment contracts (although most managers do not have such contracts) or because of the bylaws of the organization, such as membership on certain hospital board committees or on the board itself. In responding to physicians who want what you perceive to be inappropriate special considerations, you can often rely on other physicians who agree with you to see to it that such claims can be safely discounted so long as you are following appropriate procedures.

A major source of your power in dealing with physicians is that you are paid to manage and not to do anything else. You have the time and the resources to carefully and thoroughly document your opinions and positions. Your major weakness is that you are greatly outnumbered by physicians, who control the production process and who have legitimate interests in joining together to oppose management and other organizational or external groups.

An example of antimanagerial cooperative behavior among physicians is reflected in Item 5, Chapter 11, in which Alexander Greenspan, the chairman of the radiology department, complains to Victor Alan, administrator of Glory Hospital, about the insufficiency of Alan's response to claims for more and better medical equipment. Greenspan claims to be speaking on behalf of the medical staff, whether or not he has been delegated that authority. As part of his statement, Greenspan asserts, "The medical board members are charged by the hospital trustees with the professional medical operation of this hospital."

Accommodating Each Other

It may be useful to examine some specific problems that managers face in dealing with physicians. Remember, if you are trying to influence the behavior of powerful persons, it is best to focus on one or two issues at a time, rather than to attempt to institute broad initiatives in many areas.

Managers sometimes have to respond to patient or staff complaints about the poor quality of care provided by physicians. In Item 19, Chapter 11, Victor Alan receives a complaint concerning the way a patient's daughter has been treated in the emergency department. Alan refers this problem to Ivan Bolles, the chief of emergency services, who admits (Item 20, Chapter 11) that the physician on duty in the emergency department did give an improper explanation. (Bolles also indicates that he was already aware of the situation.) Bolles asks Alan to convey his apologies to the mother and to tell her that "we will do our best to prevent a similar reoccurrence."

For a second example, a board member's wife indicates to Alan that women in the community that Glory Hospital serves go out of town for obstetrical services because of the bad personal reputation of two members of the local obstetrical group. In a third example, a staff nurse informs Alan that a local osteopath visits only infrequently the patients whom he admits, calls for consultants if any problems ensue, and does not clear consultations in advance with his patients, who are unaware that their insurance does not reimburse them for such consultations.

Concerning these last two examples, administrator Alan can report the situations to an appropriate medical staff review group, speak to the physicians involved (who are unlikely to appreciate it), or do nothing. Since managers can do little to alter these situations, many managers ignore them. Problems of this kind should generally be handled by medical officials. The lack of accountability of medical officials to governing boards and to chief executive officers is, I believe, a critical problem in many health services organizations.

In communicating with physicians, stay calm, polite, and consistent unless some valid reason for acting otherwise comes up. Your tone in conversation should be steady and never patronizing. Remember that physicians want to know what behavior they can expect from you. They want you to be on their side, particularly when they are "wrong." You must attempt to do what is "right" for the patient and the payer for medical care, but you must also protect your job. Others should expect from you only what you as a manager, or what any other manager, can do in a given situation.

To work effectively with physicians, you must earn the trust of physician and governing board leaders and be an able advocate of what you wish to accomplish. Physicians must know that you take their interests into account when making decisions. You may be able to persuade physicians to give up a short-term interest now for some greater gain in the future, but often only if you can show them that not giving it up will cost them more. When physicians will not yield, you generally should. Time may eventually prove your judgment to have been sound.

Working Together: Some Examples

Three recurring problems that hospital managers and physicians face are late completion of medical records, effective decision making on capital budgeting, and development and implementation of new service programs (or abandonment of ineffective or inefficient existing service programs).

Late Completion of Medical Records

A typical problem in short-term general hospitals is completion of medical records within the specified time. According to the Accreditation Manual for Hospitals, "records of discharged patients shall be completed following discharge, within a reasonable period of time to be specified in the medical staff rules and regulations." Prompt completion of medical records may be important to a hospital's cash flow, because bills cannot be sent to third-party payers until physicians fill in their diagnoses. Often hospital medical staffs have rules stating that records must be completed within a certain number of days after discharge.

> *EXAMPLE:*
> Loss of admitting privileges is the penalty for late completion of records at Urban Community Hospital, a 250-bed general hospital affiliated with Urban HMO. About 20 percent of Urban Hospital's admissions are HMO patients. It is a fairly common practice for non-HMO physicians, many of whom have busy practices, to violate the rules and to keep admitting patients while they are "catching up" on their backlog of incomplete medical records, thus causing the hospital to lose considerable cash flow.
>
> "Why don't these physicians, like the HMO physicians, complete their medical records on time?" asks Tony Bullitt, administrator of Urban Hospital. Dr. Marshall says he is too busy taking care of patients and attending hospital committee meetings. Dr. Burns dislikes completing medical records, believing it is not really a very good use of his time. Dr. Clyde wants to know why someone else can't do more of the job or make it easier for him to complete his medical records, adding that last week the dictating equipment was broken and his wife, Thelma, was ill.

Probably there is no acceptable solution to the problem of late and incomplete medical records. Administrator Bullitt tries to see that individual physicians meet the standards of acceptable performance set by the medical staff for all admitting physicians. This may include suspending some physicians. Complete compliance with the current medical staff rules is usually not feasible and is not expected at Urban Hospital. Bullitt tells the medical records committee and offending physicians when the backlog gets particularly high or an accreditation visit draws near. He explains the nature and extent of the problem and asks the committee to make recommendations based on the medical staff rules. Bullitt supplies the committee chairman, Dr. Marshall, with information on who the chief offenders are, what the patterns of dereliction are, what this is costing the hospital, and why current sanctions are not working.

It takes some time for the medical records committee to convene and to make recommendations, which usually involve stricter enforcement of the rules. Dr. Marshall can refer problem offenders to their respective department chiefs. This approach works in an HMO because few physicians are involved and they are salaried. However, by the time Dr. Marshall talks to each department chief and the latter actually sit down and discuss the problem with the attending physicians involved (assuming the chiefs want to do this), the problem may no longer exist or the offenders may be different.

Some physicians do come in and complete charts when the head of the medical records department writes or calls them or when they receive a notice halting their admissions privileges until their charts are completed. Others may attempt to admit patients in their own name or under a partner's name if the policy is not strictly enforced.

Administrator Bullitt, in the example, does everything within his power to limit managerial or institutional contributions to the problem. He has asked the medical records department to keep an accurate accounting of the situation. With the advice of the department head and in consultation with peer managers and state hospital association consultants, Bullitt attempts to determine how much of the problem Urban Hospital can tolerate, given other constraints. Bullitt also works through the medical staff executive committee to improve physician performance. He documents what he has tried to do about any hospital contributions to the problem. If all else fails (and Bullitt is certain that the organization can no longer tolerate the current performance of certain physicians), Bullitt discusses the problem with the chairman of his board. They may decide to wait before bringing the matter before the hospital joint conference committee.

What Bullitt does not do is harass the offending physicians or complain about them and Dr. Marshall's medical records committee to physician and board leaders. Rather, at the next board finance committee meeting, Bullitt tells the committee what impact the late records are having on hospital cash flow. Bullitt has been careful not to blame the head of the medical records department for failing to ensure physician compliance. Bullitt has insisted that the department head provide him with accurate reporting, that the department staff be pleasant to physicians, and that the department head occasionally bend the rules, particularly when the hospital is to blame or when a usually conscientious physician is overcome by other responsibilities and circumstances.

After the finance committee meeting and before the accreditation visit, a mutual accommodation has been reached at Urban Hospital. All late records have been completed. In the process, physicians have gotten a better understanding of the importance of meeting the standards, while managers have gotten a better understanding of some of the problems physicians face in completing their records promptly.

Capital Budgeting

EXAMPLE:
At Highsmith Hospital, administrator Cal Calderone asks all physician chiefs and nonmedical department heads to make equipment requests for the next three years and to classify requests as (1) emergent (for medical care reasons or because they are required by licensing and accrediting authorities) or money-saving; (2) important and needed; and (3) nice to have. Category 3 is

useful for requesters so that they will not forget to put these items on the list again the next year, perhaps in category 2. Physician chiefs and department heads are asked to validate or document their priority requests. In what ways, if any, does the requested equipment produce greater benefits or result in lower costs as compared with present equipment, if applicable?

While this budgetary process rumbles on, and some physicians never adequately justify certain requests (which does not mean they lack priority), Calderone and his vice-president for financial affairs, Kevin Murphy, attempt to estimate the funds that will be available next year for buying or leasing capital equipment. This amount is never precise, because the hospital can always spend a little more and often should spend a little less; there must also be a sufficient reserve available to meet contingencies. Another problem Calderone faces is how to develop valid (to the requesting physician, other chiefs, and management) criteria for allocating capital funds between medical (not always easy to define) and nonmedical requests.

Calderone and Murphy come up with a range of recommended spending amounts, by category, for the next year. Meanwhile, the executive committee of the medical staff has come up with its equipment list, which totals substantially more than the finance committee of the board of trustees (and Calderone and Murphy) wishes to spend. At this point, a fund-raising drive can be considered to fill in the gap: so what if some of the surgical equipment purchased last year has only been used once or twice? Will the physicians kick in for new medical equipment* if the funds cannot be raised in the community or from donors? Should they?

Murphy suggests to Calderone a more-or-less rational procedure for capital budgeting. First, create an effective finance committee of the governing board, to include physician members with clout among their peers; this committee will develop limits for capital expenditures, based on some percentage of hospital gross or net revenues. Document the extent to which equipment purchases have been justified. Develop criteria in the department of financial affairs for the medical staff to consider in making capital budgeting decisions. Provide adequate support staff to the physician chiefs to assist in equipment justification.

Calderone points out to Murphy some of the things that can go wrong with such a more-or-less rational approach. First, the finance committee is comprised of trustees who do not wish to set or to adhere to strictly specified standards. Second, it would be political suicide for Murphy or Calderone to make public capital expenditures that did not prove to be justified. Third, the medical staff may not agree on the criteria used to evaluate capital expenditures or may refuse to set priorities after a certain amount in excess requests has been lopped off. Fourth, Murphy's staff and physician chiefs may lack the time and the will to develop comprehensive justifications for certain desired equipment within the given time, and Calderone will not approve extra staff for the department of financial affairs to do it.

----

* Some hospitals have instituted mandatory plans for physician "contributions." For such a proposed plan, see Item 14, Chapter 11.

From a political perspective, Calderone does not want to give certain physicians the opportunity to single him out as the reason why their equipment requests are being denied, especially if rival physicians' requests are being honored. He suggests that the board consider establishing dollar ceilings related to the amount external payers will allow. He asks the board chairman to recommend that the board and the medical staff set and approve criteria for evaluating capital expenditure requests. Murphy's staff can assist chiefs in justifying future requests. As long as the medical staff participates in the allocation process, due process will be observed; and if the governing board sets a limit on the amount to be spent on medical equipment, Calderone feels that the capital budgeting process will be acceptable to most physicians. Whether there will be enough money to fund a sufficient amount of desired and agreed-upon equipment requests is, of course, another matter.

Establishing New Services

The difficulty of implementing decisions that are in the organization's interest (as defined by board members) but not in certain physician's interest should be clear by now. Board members can seldom marshall the necessary knowledge, will, and time, even with managerial support, to oppose a united group of physicians.

EXAMPLE:

Hospital administrator Victor Alan wishes to start a day care program at Glory Hospital. He believes that there is a community need (which researchers at a nearby Eastern University are eager to validate), that start-up funds can be raised from philanthropic sources, and that operational funds can be gotten from some third-party payers. Objections to the program are raised by Dr. Riggio, the president of the medical staff, speaking on behalf of several staff physicians. "What's the hurry in getting the university in to study the need for this program? They are going to make us look bad, accuse us of overhospitalizing our patients. We don't agree with their methodology. Who needs this program anyway? Is the hospital planning to go into competition for these patients with the medical staff? We need to spend more money on medical equipment. The hospital doesn't belong in long-term care anyway. Frankly, if this program does well, some of the guys think you, Victor Alan, as the administrator, are going to get too powerful."

Mutual accommodation between physicians and managers may mean dropping this program at this time. It is generally unwise for managers to attempt to change the goals of a direct service organization whose production process is controlled by physicians whom the manager does not control. With physician support, or at least lacking intensive physician opposition, however, some not-for-profit hospitals have started day care programs similar to the one Alan proposes.

Faced with a similar opportunity to open a new service (and thereby change the hospital's mission), many managers in the for-profit hospital corporation would not be similarly constrained, because, according to Zuckerman, "the distance of a corporate level management group provides a buffer or protection for the local administrator." In this case, the main constraints are likely to be financial. Will the new service or program be self-supporting? Many new chronic care programs, although needed, are not likely to be self-sustaining or to generate rates of return as high as those of alternative investments.

The manager of a governmental hospital, faced with a similar opportunity, may have greater difficulty in raising the necessary start-up funds or in convincing elected officials that taxpayers would be willing to finance the program. Even if the new program can be funded externally, say by a private foundation, elected officials may believe that the probability of eventually having to cut back on services or close the program when funds run out does not make its initiation worthwhile.

Investing and Spending Political Capital

EXAMPLE:
Administrator Victor Alan has spent a great deal of his scarce political capital with the Glory Hospital medical staff by (1) speaking against a candidate for the board of trustees favored by Dr. Riggio, the president of the medical staff; (2) defending Lydia Bailey, the director of nursing, who was under attack by Dr. Riggio; (3) urging a hospital day care program and a related research program documenting its need; and (4) hiring a new osteopathic chief of emergency services during the summer, without lengthy consultation with and discussion by all medical staff who wanted to be involved.

Alan's successor, Tim Collins, builds scarce political capital with the same medical staff by (1) not suggesting any new nontechnology-oriented service programs; (2) allowing radiologists to bill patients directly rather than receiving a percentage of gross revenues from the hospital; (3) giving unqualified support to medical staff requests for new diagnostic equipment; and (4) staying out of all decisions about board membership and hospital committee chairmen.

Alan, who may be a better manager in hospitals where medical staff leaders are less opposed to programmatic change, is not as effective a manager at Glory Hospital as Collins, who takes medical staff goals as a given, yet can do an effective job within these constraints for patients and the community.

Many physicians find it difficult to completely trust managers. Managers must try, therefore, to be seen as predictable and well-disposed toward physicians. Getting physicians to regard you in this way is usually, like so many other things, the result of a great deal of hard work. You must invest in relationships by helping physicians solve their problems as they see them in ways that they find helpful.

To repeat, start by doing those aspects of your job that physicians think you should be doing. It is of great advantage if the skills and talents you possess are perceived by physicians and owners or trustees as central to the organization's mission. In a hospital, such a skill can be expertise in cost reimbursement; in an HMO, marketing expertise with large groups; in the neighborhood health center, the obtaining of government grants; in the group practice, day-to-day administration.

Physicians make your job difficult by wanting things that you, as a manager, cannot supply. When physicians own the organization, as in a group practice, they may be less likely to make such demands because they are spending their own money rather than other people's. In the for-profit multihospital corporation, the physicians may not consider it appropriate to demand as much.

In certain health services organizations, it may be difficult to find any stable coalition among physicians, governing boards, community groups, unions, affiliated institutions, and regulatory officials. The manager's primary political task in such situations may be to avoid being identified with any particular power group. The manager will want to be seen by all groups as trustworthy and the most helpful contributor to the organization's effectiveness.

Political skills can be central to managerial advancement and job security. Some politicians run election campaigns by trying hard not to offend any important group and by being vague about key issues, hoping that different constituent groups will perceive them as having a position not too unlike their own. Good politicians are always in touch with their public. They are good listeners. They do favors for people, or at least respond to requests. They ask about the family, remember names and faces, send cards and flowers, and make hospital visits to constituents. This can be gruelling and demanding work, but each contact with a constituent can be educational as well. Many politicians (and managers) enjoy spending a great deal of time with people.

Suppose you are nice to many physicians, work long hours, do not encroach upon the medical staff's territory, and meet the demands made on you by your superior or external agencies. Then why are you under political attack from individual physicians or the medical staff? What can go wrong for the hardworking, pleasant-looking, attentive manager-politician?

There may be too many important physicians to please. Some physicians will not easily take no for an answer, nor will they tolerate indefinite delay. When physicians ask you for something that you cannot supply, obviously you should make sure that you really cannot get it for them. If you do some things for certain physicians, this does not always mean that you can behave similarly toward all physicians. Preferential treatment may not be fair and will be resented. But organizations are not democracies, and not all physicians contribute equally to the organization.

If you cannot give physicians what they want, see if what they want is somebody else's problem. If the chief of radiology wants an additional X-ray technician, perhaps the state rate-setting agency or the hospital's finance committee will not allow it. Do not tell the chief that other hospitals can staff the same service with fewer technicians or that his department head is a bad manager and that he, the chief, has a lousy personality. The chief sees your job as getting him what he needs, not as showing him why he does not need it: he has already made up his mind about that.

As a manager, you are often faced with the problem of "doing the right thing" (for the organization, for patients, for taxpayers) when physicians want to allocate scarce organizational resources in some way other than what you deem appropriate or acceptable. It is easier to deal with physician opposition to planned expenditures that assist the organization financially but that do not help them personally than it is to turn down their requests for new equipment or staff when rival physicians are obtaining them. If physicians see that other physicians are not getting equally needed requests, they may accept a policy of delay for awhile. Do not suggest taking away physicians' space, staff, or funds, since they regard what they already have as immutable. Do not attempt to start new services without cooperation from physicians; new ventures, because they are new, are likely to be risky anyway.

On the other hand, nothing succeeds like success. Without risk, there is no gain. There is nothing quite like obtaining new resources for an organization or providing new services to patients, especially when predecessors and competitors have been unable to acquire or provide them.

Success can also be attained by taking over an organization in a political and financial shambles and restoring order to it. This is less difficult to accomplish if you set conditions before accepting the new position and reach out to key physicians and others who may reconsider past political conflict in the face of a worsening financial situation.

Managers earn political capital by removing obstacles to physicians in their daily work. Although some physicians may see this as what you should have been accomplishing already, others will give you credit for it if you can help them better than they were being helped before. Try to be always available and not to irritate important physicians. This may be difficult, especially because some physicians may distrust attractive, pleasant, hardworking managers who are always around but who have no authority to make decisions.

Managerial success should be shared. If you take large risks, you are likely to fail often, so spread "success" and the credit for it. Likewise, share the risk. Physicians can assist you in obtaining resources for the organization that will also increase their incomes or make their work easier. Physicians can do much of the persuading and implementing related to policy change. Why not let them help, assist them to help, and let them take the credit? Physicians can help restore order when there has been political conflict and can advise the new manager as to what should be done and how it can best be accomplished. Seek out the controversial and contributing physicians for ideas and the respected and elected physician officials for advice concerning implementation. Remember, of course, that no one will be looking out for your political welfare.

Do not worry that physicians will be shy about telling you which obstacles to their work you should remove. In a hospital, these may range from firing the director of nursing to increasing the size of the physicians' parking lot. Physicians may or may not be shy about telling you to stay out of their business. When you rub physicians the wrong way, some of them will say, "Give the manager a chance;" others will wait and see which way the wind is blowing. When disaster strikes, you will usually have been given warning in the form of withdrawn contact, lessened courtesy or increased formality, or open hostility.

Having trustees, department heads, and influential persons in the community speak well of you may not create favor with physicians. Their question is often, "How well can I do with this person relative to some other manager?" They will tend to base their answer on your past behavior and on what they know about other managers. They may not know much about management, but they will have definite ideas about what it takes to make or keep the organization what they want it to be.

Your political capital can be spent in one shot, for example when physicians hear from someone else something personally negative that you have said about them. Political capital can not be regained so quickly, and building political capital is a slow and tedious process; it is done day by day, hour by hour through your managerial persistence, discipline, expertise, and luck.

Life on the Physician-Dominated Committee

An important part of the health services manager's job is serving on medical staffs or hospital committees that are dominated by physicians.

EXAMPLE:
Phil Redding, assistant administrator at Glory Hospital, has been assigned by Victor Alan to serve on the medical staff recruitment committee. The physicians on the committee include Bill McKenna, a young internist and chairman; Steve Stromboli, another internist; Lou Arfus, an obstetrician; and Bill Brown, chief of pathology. On the agenda of the committee is the recruitment of a neurosurgeon and two general practitioners. The first committee

meeting is scheduled for 8:00 a.m. Redding arrives at 8:00 a.m., McKenna at 8:05, and Stromboli and Arfus by 8:30, when the meeting begins; Brown arrives at 8:45.

McKenna reviews past attempts to recruit a neurosurgeon and how difficult it has been because of the shortage of neurosurgeons, the amount of malpractice insurance required for the specialty, and the lack of coverage, because the hospital patient load is sufficient to support only one neurosurgeon. Recruitment is hampered by the presence of an inferior neurosurgeon at a neighboring hospital and by Glory Hospital's not yet having obtained a CAT scanner. Stromboli suggests that someone attend the next national neurosurgery meeting and that the hospital advertise in the appropriate medical journals. McKenna asks Stromboli to prepare a recruitment plan, with specifics, for the next meeting.

Regarding general practice, McKenna says that the hospital governing board would guarantee one year's income to each of two new physicians. Board members have indicated that some people in town have experienced difficulty lately in obtaining a regular physician. Arfus says that he is unaware of any physician shortage and that no one guaranteed him an income when he started practice; he leaves for the operating room. Redding points out that other hospitals in the area have guaranteed first year incomes to physicians; it cost one hospital less than $10,000 last year, and the hospital's occupancy was improved. Stromboli says that doesn't mean it will happen here. "I am still taking new patients. Aren't you, Bill?" McKenna replies, "Yes, on a limited basis, but I have restricted my practice to gastroenterology." Stromboli says that he has to leave the meeting. Brown says to Redding, "Keep up the good work, Phil," as he gets up to leave the meeting. McKenna then says to Redding, "Well, that went over like a lead balloon. Let's see what happens at the next meeting."

It may be difficult for managers to get things done on such a committee and still survive politically. But committees are not always set up to get things done, at least not to get done what managers think "the organization" wants them to do. Physicians do not necessarily serve on committees because they want to get things done or even because they want to block potential changes that may threaten their interests. Physicians may feel obliged to serve on some committees, or they may simply want to know what is going on. One of the advantages of committees, from a managerial point of view, is that many of the physicians who must participate in important policy decisions will become involved in them early on. Discussing problems and alternatives with these persons can help avoid premature or mistaken attempts at policy adoption or implementation.

Some committees are interdisciplinary and focus on particular issues or problems. Standing committees, such as hospital committees on medical infections or finance, deal with recurring and important problems. Committees may also be set up on a temporary basis—for example, a hospital building subcommittee for constructing a new satellite health center, or an HMO marketing committee for enrolling the telephone workers.

Why don't committees accomplish more? Some committees function as much to test, weigh, and refine proposals as they do to plan and implement change. If change is not perceived by almost every committee member as necessary, then it may be necessary not to change. Common problems in committee functioning are as follows: (1) often no mandate or set of objectives for the committee has been formulated; (2) even if given a mandate, the committee or its chairman may not be held accountable for failing to exercise it; (3) the chairman or certain members of the committee may lack commitment to its goals or to the group process; and (4) the committee may suffer from ineffective staff work.

When conditions are favorable, there is little you have to do or should do to make committees effective, other than attending meetings, preparing and distributing staff work, helping to define issues, analyzing the consequences of specific recommendations, and documenting committee proceedings. Managers are seldom chairmen of hospital medical staff or governing board committees, but they may participate in the selection of committee chairmen, the naming of committee members, and the development of reporting and accountability systems.

Committees should usually define problems or validate the governing body's definition of problems before recommending solutions. Staff work can be done only for a limited number of solutions to a limited number of problems during a specified time. It helps if all committee members agree that there is a problem, that certain consequences are liable to result from the problem, and that the organization should do something about it.

The next step is gathering data about the extent and consequences of the problem and the costs and benefits of various solutions or approaches to it. It would be wonderful if the committee could agree at this point upon a plan whose costs of implementation were acceptable. If the committee cannot, the problem can always be, and sometimes is, reformulated or referred back for redefinition to the body that established the committee. Staff can be asked to specify, in light of new information, new alternative solutions and their costs and benefits. Whatever staff does, someone may ask for more data, and someone else may suggest that the problem is not that important after all or that this is not really the right committee to attack the problem now.

To obtain reasonable consensus among committee members, particularly on controversial subjects, it may be necessary for committee chairmen and others to lobby committee members before meetings. Generally, it is not a good idea to lobby only certain members. If the proposal is controversial and is opposed by other members and their constituents, committee recommendations may be derailed by the group that established the committee. Trying to railroad a measure through the committee may generate considerable and unnecessary antagonism among members. An important issue may thus be tabled—not because of disagreement as to its importance, but because of lack of trust in the leadership that is proposing solutions.

Committee meetings are opportunities for managers to accomplish their own objectives, too. Physicians may be available in committee meetings, or before and after such meetings, to discuss business and personal matters in a more relaxed setting than generally prevails. (Too relaxed a setting may cause problems in committee efficiency, if not effectiveness: for example, physicians may leave the room frequently to take or make telephone calls, or they may grab the telephone in the room and talk into it, sometimes loudly.) However, if you are not properly prepared for a committee meeting, engaging in last-minute private conversations with members before the meeting is likely to generate distrust. Most committee members like to feel that there is only one committee and that they are all equal members of it, not that there is a subcommittee which is really making the decisions and that they are expected to be simply rubber stamps.

Goal-oriented managers often have great difficulty controlling their behavior when a committee seems to be "going nowhere" or going "in the wrong direction." If you speak up in distress at these times, you may occasion hostility from physicians or others who disagree with what you want the committee to do. Remind yourself that, in terms of your relationships with physicians, how you behave is as important as what you do or say. If prior understandings about what the committee should produce and when, exist, you can help the chairman by validating and documenting these understandings. If prior understandings do not exist, you will not help matters by attempting to focus discussion or influence opinions. Further, it is not sufficient in such situations to be aggressively silent. You should take care to appear amiable so that physicians will not think you are displeased with them, or that you think the meeting of the committee is not very good, or that you think the committee lacks effective leadership, all of which may be true.

Part Three

Documents from the Field

A cardinal rule for the researcher is that whenever he himself feels most dubious about an important interpretation—or foresees that readers may well be dubious—then he should specify quite explicitly upon what kind of data his interpretation rests.

Barney G. Glaser and *Anselm Strauss*

IX
Maxims for Managers

When you're talkin' you're not learnin'.

Ramsey Clark

According to Karl Weick, "Aphorisms can move inquiry along; they can help people see facets of problems that they hadn't seen before. They can force people to keep asking questions, possibly improving the quality of questions that get asked, and they have the obvious advantage of honesty." In the maxims that follow, I have borrowed freely from others and summed up some of what I have learned from the mistakes I have made as a manager. The list is not meant to be exhaustive, but it does focus on some common and important problems that inexperienced—and some not-so-inexperienced—managers create for themselves.

People Are Rational When
They Disagree with You

There is always a reason why something is being done the way it is. Before changing it, consider why it was done that way in the first place and who benefits from doing it that way. Next, consider what will happen to whom if things are done the way you suggest and how you will be perceived by others if you attempt to overcome their resistance. Does this mean you should never try to change things unless everyone else agrees? No. By the time everyone else agrees, a new approach may be called for.

Beware of dividing people into "good guys," who agree with you, and "bad guys," who disagree with you. For one thing, the "bad guys" would not be a problem if they did not have powerful protectors or if you were not dependent on them or their allies. Maybe they are really good guys and you are just in their way. Persons who oppose you are likely to know why they oppose you—and it will not be simply because you represent "progress." One thing is certain: if the change you seek is made over their objections and they are bad guys after all, they are going to see to it that your idea does not work—and that you do not work, either.

One approach to making changes that sometimes works is to confront your opponents with the problem. Ask them to solve it. Then tell them what is right with their solutions.

Don't Fear the Vestedness of Their Interests,
Fear That You Haven't Done Your Homework

Be prepared when someone asks, "How is your idea going to work?" You have to know better than anyone else how it is going to work, what might go wrong with it, and what the chances are that it will go wrong. Before implementing ideas that were successful elsewhere, be sure you have tailored them to fit your organization.

In most health services organizations, the most powerful persons are the owners or trustees and the key physicians, who can veto your proposals to help patients or broaden organizational mission. Worry about doing your homework rather than about physicians or others opposing you. If you have done your homework and they oppose you, at least you were not derelict in doing your job. If you have not done your homework, you should be discharged for wasting everybody's time—even if yours was a good idea that would have worked in the organization and people are only opposed to it because they do not understand it. Failure will be forgotten once and forgiven twice. The third time, look to your references and your resume.

If Management Doesn't Make a Difference,
What Are You Doing, Anyway?

Respect your position, for without it you would not have a job. Could the work you do be divided up and shared by other managers and nonmanagers? Does much of your work have to be done at all?

What are the most important and the second most important aspects of your job? How well do you do them? Do you spend too much, just enough, or not enough time on the most important functions? Does everybody know what you are contributing? Do the key participants or stakeholders know? What new resources have you obtained for the organization lately?

Are you seen by physicians and board members as helpful, even if not critical, to the organization? Do they see what you do as valuable or potentially valuable to them, or do they see you as a threat, a nullity, or an obstruction? You can make them perceive you as valuable by being cheerful, respectful, and considerate and by consulting with them both before you make decisions that will affect them and after, during implementation. You want to be able to tell them in advance which of the promises you made you may not be able to keep because of changed circumstances. All this consulting takes considerable time, which means you will not be able to accomplish as much as you might like to. So what? No matter how much you accomplish, more remains to be done. You will benefit from investing in relationships with powerful people; and, if you do your homework, making and implementing the next smart decision will take less time and go more smoothly.

*Ask Yourself What People Want,
Not How You Feel about Them*

Assume that you have a fixed amount of time in which to deal with persons whose work interacts with yours. When you spend time with some people, you are not spending time with others. How are the others going to feel about your not spending enough time with them or too much time with somebody else?

There is an old saying that managers should not get too close to their ballplayers. People compliment you, are pleasant to you, and use your time because they want something from you. There is nothing wrong with this: you are doing the same thing, otherwise you would not have gotten where you are.

It is not enough to remember that people will use you. How others perceive the persons who they think are using you may be just as important. Whatever you do with your favorites, even if you do not know that they are your favorites, will be interpreted by others to your disadvantage. Do people become your favorites by making above-average contributions to organizational effectiveness, or do they get where they are primarily by flattery?

It Is Better to Say "No" than "Maybe"

Always request a day in which to think about a claim, demand, or request: never answer right away. If you say no, you can always reconsider, and the claimants will be grateful. If you say yes and then reconsider, claimants will feel that you have taken something away from them and they will bear a grudge.

Get your part of the bargain agreed to first: no bargaining is possible with persons who are more powerful than you. Sometimes you cannot give people what they want because you do not have it to give, perhaps because a third party, more powerful than you, is opposed. Always assume that, if you give someone something he or she should not have, everyone else will know about it, and immediately.

*If You Aren't Prepared When Opportunity Knocks,
It May Pass You By—
Or, Worse Yet, You May Grab It*

Plan for your next job now; that way, if someone asks you to take on more responsibility, you can begin thinking about the terms on which you would accept the offer.

The same thinking applies to accomplishment in your job. Stockpile ideas and plans so that when extra funds are available you will be prepared to take advantage of them. It is never a waste of time to develop plans and strategies; the process may help you determine what it is really possible for you to do now.

Consider how a proposed job change would affect your life-style and that of your family. Is your salary adequate now? What will the added stress and time at work entailed in a new job mean for you and your family?

Before accepting new responsibilities, know yourself and attempt to discover why you are being offered them. Is it because you have been effectively discharging your current responsibilities? If so, is there good reason to think that the players and the rules of the new game will be similar? Do not move before you are ready, unless you are willing to risk failure. Most of you have 40 to 45 years to work, so why rush to change a situation you were more or less happy with before you received the new offer?

If You Aren't Allowed to Do
What You Want To Do,
Focus upon What You Can Do

In any job there will be decisions that you consider right and appropriate, based upon the long-range interests of the organization's clientele or the intentions of its founders, but that are not timely. Owners, trustees, and physicians may perceive your contribution to the organizational welfare primarily in terms of your contribution to their own good, which may or may not coincide with what you consider to be the organizational welfare. But there is so much to be done to benefit patients and to support physicians, nurses, and others, why not get to work?

Do not blow your own trumpet too loudly or urge everyone else to make changes your way rather than their way. Results, not just working hard, are the desired contribution.

You should always have more to do than you can possibly accomplish. This does not always mean that you should do more work, only that you can always keep yourself fully occupied. There is joy in working well, but there is also joy in not having to rush everyone. Limit your time in the office: most of you are more dispensable at work than at home. Limit your thinking about work at home: it will make you a more interesting person. When you are working, however, focus your effort and concentrate on what is important. Be prepared to work extra hours, but only as appropriate.

Never Say Behind Someone's Back
Anything You Wouldn't Say to His Face

There is a difference between speaking ill of what someone is doing and speaking ill of the person. If you are envious of or opposed to the person's policy, it is a sign of weakness to have to speak against him or her in personal terms. Besides, the person to whom you are speaking may be the other person's friend or may agree with his or her policy and not with yours.

There is an indirect way of speaking ill of others, by making statements about them in a tone that can only be interpreted negatively. "Did you know that person X has been married three times, has a house in Shelter Island, has a son who is homosexual?" and so forth. Or, "Did you know person Y plays tennis Wednesday afternoons, eats at expensive restaurants at organizational expense, gives his secretary Thursday mornings off to see her psychiatrist?" Does telling someone else this kind of stuff do you any good, or are you spending valuable time worrying about what someone else is making or doing, what their friends are doing, how much they work, or whatever?

This does not mean that you should not ask questions about other people or listen to what others say about people. You do need to know a lot about the people whose performance you depend on, but what you need to know is what they expect from you, how they perceive you, and what their strengths and limitations are. What people are saying about others can also be important because the speakers' feelings may affect work relationships. As a rule, however, you should counter negative comments about others with positive comments or validating questions such as "Are you really sure?" "That isn't what I've observed," or "So what, he does a good job around here."

A related point is that you gain nothing by revealing yourself. Others will not necessarily reveal themselves because of it. Have respect for your position. School yourself to talk in pleasantries: even the weather can be really interesting if you are focusing upon building a relationship rather than having a meaningful dialogue. When you reveal yourself you are defining yourself, and that gives someone else a reason to dislike you. Further, you are showing favoritism to the person whom you tell. Maybe the somebody else they tell your revelation to does not own something you own, does not have kids as smart as your kids. And they resent it. What others do not know about you will not hurt you.

By the Time You Are Really Unhappy
in Your Present Job, You May Not Have
Adequate Time for a Job Search

Most managers do not stay with the same health services organization throughout their careers. Reasons for changing jobs include blocked advancement, the wish to try something new, a new boss with whom you do not want to work, and a new boss who is dissatisfied with your work.

You will probably begin to think of leaving your present job long before you are actually ready to do so, and you will probably stay at your present job for awhile after you have decided that you are ready to move. Plan for moving well enough in advance to give yourself sufficient flexibility to respond to an appropriate opportunity and to accept largely on your own terms. Using a new offer to raise your current compensation is generally not wise. If your boss knows you are thinking of leaving, he or she may start thinking about replacing you.

You should be thinking frequently about what it is you want in a job, and you should be establishing and maintaining a network of acquaintances who can help you get where you want to be. At the same time, you must be producing results in your present position. Your boss's recommendation is always important. You can leave on friendly terms by having produced results and by not having asked the boss continually for something the boss could not give.

Establishing and maintaining a network of acquaintances can help you in your present job, and it should be enjoyable. "Doing favors" for other people includes listening to what they are saying, not just offering yourself through them to all potential employers. At the same time, you want some of your acquaintances to be people who can help you. There is not much you can do for well-established powerful people in return except be grateful, but that may be enough if you knew them before you were asking for a favor. If you strain to do something for someone of higher status, and the effort is inappropriate, it may not be appreciated. Seek out effective managers, and seek the advice and assistance of experienced and respected mentors, some of whom may now be out of the mainstream of health services management. Their advice and judgment may be useful to you in deciding what to do, as well as in finding a specific job. Consider what they are telling you and let them know whether you intend to follow their advice. Let them know, too, how things turn out.

When Someone Attacks You,
He Isn't Telling You Everything

If others attack you publicly, try not to respond immediately. Later, ask them to explain what was on their minds. What was behind what they were saying? Did they mean what you thought they meant? Were they responding to something they thought you said, and was that what you had intended to say? If not, say so. And you should not attack anyone more powerful than you openly or unexpectedly. This is sufficient reason for a boss to discharge you. If you are the boss, corporate life is difficult enough without having someone who is supposedly on your side be publicly disloyal.

Try to understand why people may dislike and fear you. Being disliked and feared is never going to do you any good unless you are top dog and powerful enough to remain so. You will be disliked if you are seen by powerful persons as not being one of them by virtue of your occupation, age, sex, education, race, ethnic group, or whatever. Some persons may think that you do not listen to them or appreciate them, that you play favorites, or that you do not take their views into account. They may find you inconsiderate, obese, depressing, or immoral. Do not give anyone an unnecessary reason for disliking you; the policies you advocate may be reason enough.

If others dislike your policies and wish to dislike you, they can find ample justification: you are too modest, formal, proper, cheerful for their tastes. These traits, however, may be what your position calls for and what others value in you. Uncommitted persons in the organization are more likely to rally to your defense if they do not find your behavior threatening, unpredictable, or inappropriate.

Those Who Have Helped You Will Help You Again; as for Those Who Have Hurt You, . . .

The amazing thing about human nature is not that there are so many brutish people, but that there are so many kindly people. There may be no way for you to pay kindly people back except by being kind to persons who are dependent on you. When you ask persons who have helped you once to help you again, they do. What they have to give is not always what you want to receive, but their listening can help you refocus your thinking, plans, and action. Never surrender your judgment completely to anyone, but remember that you can further inform your judgment by responding genuinely to others' questions and concern.

When others speak ill of you, or do not give you a chance, or oppose you on principle, your aim must be to ignore them, not to respond to them, not to ask them for anything, and not to expect anything from them. They are unlikely to tell you the real reasons they dislike or despise you; they are unlikely even to admit to you that they dislike or despise you. Being kind to those who have hurt you is only going to be interpreted as weakness or stupidity.

On the other hand, you will be the one who suffers if you seek revenge against those who have hurt you. It could breed more trouble, and, most important, feeling and expressing anger will distract you from the important work you have to do.

Don't Expect from Others Something You Aren't Doing Yourself

Unrealistic expectations are as bad as overpromising. If you expect the impossible, it is only just that you be denied the possible. By all means have high expectations of yourself. Work hard and well. The successful manager works harder and more intelligently than the competition. This is what you want to encourage in those who work with you and for you.

Do not ask from others what you do not have or do not contribute yourself. This does not mean that others have to do a job the same way you would do it—individuals have different strengths and weaknesses. It should not surprise you when your peers and subordinates do some of their tasks or perform some of their roles better than you can or do. This is as it should be, particularly when all of you share some of the same values, can appreciate each others' differences, and respect each others' talents and contributions.

X
Interview with a Hospital Administrator: Norman Urmy, May 13, 1981

The chance to do well by doing good is the double lure of health care administration.

Suzanne Seixas

At the time this interview was conducted Norman Urmy was vice-president of New York University Medical Center and administrator of University Hospital, a 726-bed teaching hospital in New York City. After graduating from Williams College, he received his master's degree from the school of business at the University of Chicago. He has worked for 12 years at New York University Medical Center, progressing from administrative assistant to assistant administrator, associate administrator, administrator, and chief executive officer of University Hospital. Mr. Urmy is currently executive director of Vanderbilt University Hospital in Nashville, Tennessee.

How did you decide to become a hospital administrator?

After experimentation. I was a premed dropout, something I have learned is not that uncommon in the hospital administration field. My father, a physician, suggested that I consider the field, although I'm not sure just how much he knew about the job he was recommending. I got a job as a clerk in the emergency room at the Massachusetts General Hospital and spent a year there. While there, I spoke several times with a few of the administrators and, as a result of the experience, ended up applying to a number of graduate programs in hospital administration. I was accepted at the University of Chicago. The summer between my two academic years, I was placed in an "administrative residency" at University Hospital. The administrator offered me a job as an administrative assistant, which I accepted, and upon graduation I went to work at University Hospital. I remained tentative about the field until after receiving my MBA and getting into my first job.

What do hospital administrators do?

The primary function of a hospital administrator is to provide integration and coordination within the hospital. A hospital consists of a multitude of

---

This interview has been included to get the perspective of a younger manager whom I admire and who has a background different from mine. Mr. Urmy is eight years my junior, attended school in the midwest, and worked for many years in the same hospital, a large teaching institution.

highly specialized subgroups, each of which has a legitimate and different focus on the business of hospital care. Hospital administration's function is to coordinate and integrate all of these diverse perspectives into a coordinated and unified delivery of patient services. All of this must be done while keeping the delivery of these services effective clinically as well as efficient and cost-effective.

The way this integration occurs is by getting consensus among these groups. This means meetings and talking with people. Hospital administration is definitely not an activity where a single person sits in isolation and pulls strings or makes big decisions. You are dealing with people who have diverse, often competing, interests across a broad spectrum of skills and educational backgrounds. The hardest part of the job is to act as a catalyst for change while holding these interest groups together and, at the same time, keeping broad institutional goals and issues in focus. This is what many call leadership and direction. Because of the great number of interest groups and the varying degrees of power each holds, it is impossible to survive as an administrator without performing this integrative function. That is why consensus is so important in hospital management. Occasionally there are executive decisions, but they are the exception rather than the rule.

The work is both frustrating and exciting—frustrating because it takes a long time and a lot of effort to reach consensuses. You don't go home every night counting your accomplishments. Although I may have gone to six meetings and put in a ten-hour day, I sometimes feel I didn't get anything done. There are often conflicting goals, which require negotiation and trade-offs. You've got to be able to deal with that or you won't like this kind of work. Compromise is very much a part of the job. In addition, there is a high degree of external regulation of hospitals, particularly in states like New York. Such regulation limits options and creates problems in and of itself. Dealing with the regulatory environment is a challenge. Hospital administration is problems and challenges.

What do you like about your job?

I like the constant variety, dealing with intelligent, interesting, and committed people. I face challenges which are real, and when I do accomplish something, it is very exciting and satisfying—probably because significant accomplishment is so difficult. There is, however, plenty of opportunity to make a significant contribution to organizational performance. Evidence of this is that, under the same economic and political environments and constraints, certain hospitals are able to operate in the black while others are not. Even with all the competing forces, diverse interest groups, and heavy regulations, there is room to maneuver and to accomplish significant advances.

What don't you like about your job?

For me, the frustration is the most difficult part of the job. I'm extremely goal-oriented, a trait, by the way, that I think you have to have in this business. For the reasons I stated before, accomplishment is not easy. Sometimes I don't like the politics, either. In retrospect, I realize we don't always do what's best or right for the patients that we're serving. I don't like the degree of encroachment by third parties and regulators, although I understand the reasons why it's happened: hospitals have not paid sufficient attention to the people and the institutions who have been paying hospital bills, the state and federal governments.

What do administrators contribute to hospital effectiveness? What difference do you make?

There is definitely an opportunity to contribute to hospital effectiveness. Administrators do make a difference. We help to set up mechanisms that tend to encourage the efficient, smooth delivery of service. We can affect the quality of care, as well. For example, the tissue committee is usually intended to be the watchdog within the organization of the practice of the surgical staff. The administrator can make a difference by making sure that the committee is doing its job. He can go to the meetings and, if the committee is not functioning well or is overlooking abuses, he can do something about it by changing the membership of the committee. The administrator has to keep his finger on the pulse of the organization and keep watching for areas that require improvement. When such situations develop, it's the job of the administrator to intervene, to cause change, to force the institution to address the specific problems.

What are the differences between good and mediocre hospital administrators?

The best way to answer that question is to describe their qualities and traits. Excellent administrators command the respect of those working for them, especially the professional groups. Respect leads to credibility, and without that the administrator is ineffective. Good administrators are quick to grasp the important issues within the institution. They have to be able to relate to the problems of the various groups and be of service to them. The best administrators have good judgment and often demonstrate a commonsense approach to problems. They must be able to deal with frustration and keep many things going simultaneously. In some respects, administration is a juggling act. A key to the excellent administrator's success is his or her ability to attract high quality staff, within the administrative office as well as throughout the institution, and then to delegate responsibility and authority to that staff. It's impossible to be a good administrator without good supportive staff around you. Many administrators are afraid of this, are threatened by good staff around them. The best ones are not threatened but thrive on the challenges and stimulation from a strong staff.

Good administrators have to have some technical skills: a good basis in accounting and knowledge of computers, to mention a couple. Good administrators stay current with regulation and legislation in their area.

Finally, the best administrators take an active interest in the operation of their hospital. That means they have to understand all component parts of the hospital and how they interrelate. To do this, an administrator must know what's going on and see that production standards are being met. When you combine all that with just plain hard work, I think you're going to have a really good administrator.

How did you learn to become a hospital administrator?

I think there were four basic components in my education. A large number of my skills were learned before I knew anything about the field. I would describe this as my "life experience" prior to deciding on hospital administration as a career. I learned common sense, the ability to deal directly with people, and how to appreciate competing interests. The second phase of my education was my liberal arts undergraduate courses. In many ways an administrator has to be a generalist, and the smattering of different course material found in my liberal arts program has served me well. The third phase was my graduate education, where my efforts were highly focused on the specific issues relating to hospital management. The fourth stage has been the on-the-job training. Many technical aspects of hospital administration, as well as the ability to recognize the institutional issues and read the power-political system, were learned on the job. Also, I have modeled myself after other good administrators. These are people for or with whom I've worked and whom I've admired for their skill in various aspects of the job. Assimilating useful aspects of their style has been an important part of my career development.

What advice can you give someone in graduate school who wants to become a hospital administrator?

Generically, hospitals are businesses just like any other. Of course there are differences, but that can be said of any industry. Therefore, I would recommend to those in graduate school that they take as much of the traditional management course work as they can fit in. By this I mean accounting, systems, statistics, finance, capital investment, human-personnel relations, to mention a few. The courses specific to hospital management are useful as well, although most of what you learn in these courses can also be learned on the job. What you cannot learn on the job as easily are the basic disciplines. As the administrator, you will be working with various specialists, such as accountants, computerniks, physicians, technicians, and pharmacists. You must be able to at least know what these experts are talking about. Therefore, your course work should allow you to be familiar and comfortable with the subject matter that these experts represent.

What advice can you give an assistant administrator who wants to become an administrator?

Do well. I look for someone who has shown a progression in his work. Assistant administrators should look for, ask for various assignments. They should move around, get experience with different segments of the hospital so that they understand each. That broad base is very important, even though it may take you into areas in which you have little interest or marginal skills. Serve on different committees.

Additionally, you should engage in a regular dialogue with your boss. You should seek to be brought along on some of the matters which he or she does so that you can develop that different perspective or reference point. The administrator often has a different way of looking at things than the assistant administrator. There are bigger issues than those to which an assistant is exposed, and they must be learned. The assistant administrator will not be able to learn them all, but at least he or she should get the exposure. I think administrators are flattered when their assistants come to them for "career counseling." In addition to improving your relationship with the administrator, such sessions can be very useful in terms of defining areas that need work or exposure.

How has the field changed since you went to graduate school?

The biggest change has been the improved overall skill levels of hospital administrators. There are fewer administrators now who have worked themselves up through the ranks, the school of hard knocks. There are, instead, more graduate school products with higher education. There are also a lot more people in the field, due primarily to the phenomenal growth in the number of programs. There were about 12 such programs when I went to school; now there are over 70. This has led to incredible competition among graduates.

I think public attitudes are also very different. Hospitals are not sacred anymore. People read about mismanagement, overpaid executives, and so on. People weren't talking about cost containment when I started in the field. Now it's virtually the watchword. I think there's less room for hospitals and administrators to maneuver these days because of the heavy regulation and emphasis on cost containment. There's a much greater sense of public accountability, too. I think with the scarcer dollars for the industry and the increased accountability to those outside the institution, there's a lot more pressure and requirement for skillful management than there was 12 years ago. It's just harder to be a good administrator these days.

What are some of the important decisions you have had to make as an administrator?

Most decisions evolve out of a consensus of discussions with many different and diverse groups. There are some decisions, however, that do rest on the administrator's shoulders. One of the most important is the hiring of management staff. More than most areas, this is one where the hospital administrator has almost total discretion. I'm convinced that you should hire department heads and assistants that are as good as you are. Some administrators feel threatened by hiring such individuals, but you can influence the quality of hospital service by having good people managing it. Good people working for you make you look good. The director of nursing is perhaps the most significant of these positions and is one of the key jobs in any hospital.

Other large decisions are quite often not directly attributable to the administrator. The administrator, however, has a major influence in directing the institution toward the issues requiring or demanding decisions. In this way the administrator does influence the decisions that are made. Stated another way, the administrator controls the agenda of topics about which the organization makes decisions. A good example of this is the cooperative care unit at University Hospital. After the concept was developed, administration caused the institution to work through a decision-making process involving a host of groups and individuals. We didn't actually make the decision to proceed, but we caused that decision to be made. I think administrators may kid themselves in thinking a decision such as this one, which was a $20 million decision, is really theirs to make.

I think we get involved in making decisions to not do something as often as making decisions to proceed. Quite often after a thorough review, what seemed like a good idea at first turns out to be counterproductive or too risky. Administrators can't make decisions in a vacuum because of all the special skills and advice that are needed to institute change within a hospital. With scarce dollars the risks are greater, so the wise administrator gets input from all the affected and involved segments of the institution. The decision-making process actually turns out to be a planning process.

What kind of mistakes have you made as an administrator?
Hopefully, I'm making fewer mistakes now than I did a few years ago. One mistake I made fairly regularly early in my career was to enter into confrontation situations. I did not understand the complexity of the issues and the legitimate differences in opinion, and I tended to take opposing opinions personally. This was a natural reaction, but it can be devastating for long-term relationships. To be an effective administrator, you must maintain the trust and credibility of the hospital staff. Also, I have hired some people I shouldn't have hired and have had to go through the pain of separating them. Finally, I've made a few blunders of a financial nature. For example, I instituted an outpatient laboratory to

provide better service to patients. This lab duplicated our inpatient facility and in so doing raised overall costs more than new revenue. We didn't begin to recoup that loss until five years later.

When you hire an assistant administrator or a department head, what are you looking for?
The qualifications you are looking for are fairly straightforward. They include good technical knowledge, particularly in the area they will be working in; general management knowledge and experience; common sense; the ability to communicate; and a probability of a good organizational fit.

The best indicator of all is demonstrated success in their present job. Prior performance can be evaluated through references by administrative or medical staff contacts. Perhaps just as important is a history of promotion within their current organization. While organizations may hold on to marginally performing people, they rarely promote them, so promotion is a good indicator of a successful individual. The interview process allows you the opportunity to assess the person's ability to communicate and to assess the degree of fit of the individual to the organization. Questions the candidate asks about your organization are often telling about these two factors. Recently, when we were looking for someone to fill an assistant administrator position, one candidate's questions were about how he would work with the medical staff and the board of trustees, areas of contact that were not a likely part of the job. The person we did hire asked questions at a more appropriate level, and it was obvious that there would be a better fit with that second candidate. One final way to differentiate among candidates is the educational background. Although this is less significant when hiring an experienced individual, it is important when hiring someone for his or her first position.

What are your greatest problems as an administrator?
The two biggest problems facing an administrator are integration and coordination of services, which I've discussed before, and matching up the institution's programs with available resources. Hospital programs are defined by the patient population that is being treated. The patient population, in turn, is defined by the physicians on staff, and, generally speaking, physicians are free agents, not in the employ of the institution. The result is that the hospital has little direct control over its programs. Deciding what program should go ahead of others and which program should get resources, therefore, becomes a complicated process.

A tangential matter is that changes in institutional programs impact directly on physician incomes. Defining the mission for an institution and the strategic plans to implement that mission becomes very difficult. It's not the same as a production operation where you control your product line and you can decide how many widgets you're going to produce. Even if you define all the programs and get agreement on where you want the institution to go, implementation can be very difficult. It may involve recruiting physicians or building reputations in certain areas or markets. At our hospital we didn't have a strong medical oncology service, although we had been designated as a regional cancer center and had a large surgical oncology service. So we recruited some strong medical oncologists. They did just what we wanted; in fact, they exceeded our expectations, and now we have a "booming" medical oncology service. Program determines costs and staffing requirements, and, in an evironment in which there are severe shortages of both money and personnel (particularly nurses), they can be problematic. The challenge for the administrator is to define the equation which fits the institution's abilities and resources and then to coordinate and integrate it into existence so that you've got an efficient and effective operation.

Where do you find your greatest satisfactions?

In recognition of accomplishment. Maybe this is a function of my personality or working in a large hospital. The more we are able to accomplish, the better I feel. I think this is true of most people in this business, that is, the need for positive feedback. I enjoy putting the final touches on something so that I can say, "This is finished," which happens very rarely. It is satisfying to receive positive letters from patients and from physicians complimenting the institution.

What is different about being an administrator of a teaching hospital?

Adding the teaching component to a hospital is simply adding another dimension. It adds a few more major interest groups, such as house staff, faculty, and research scientists, which make things more complicated. Faculty and clinicians overlap, and signals are not always clear. There is legitimate conflict and competition for resources between the patient service and the educational parts of the organization. Being an educational institution means changes in patient mix, which influences program and resources. It adds layers of complexity to the manager's tasks. Services are the same, but issues become more complex. Teaching hospitals tend to be larger and more specialized than community hospitals. To me, the teaching hospital adds challenge which makes the job more interesting and rewarding in the long run.

On the positive side, a teaching hospital can provide a real ego boost. There's a certain status associated with the teaching centers. I imagine that a hospital administrator in a community hospital has to know the specifics of a lot more things. At a large hospital there are specialists in finance, purchasing, and personnel, to mention a few. The teaching hospital is a more political environment, "political" in a positive sense.

What is different about being a hospital administrator in New York City?
I think New York just adds a layer of pressure which is not found in many other settings. New Yorkers want to be first in everything and to be the most sophisticated. This is what I call the New York City effect, and it raises the level of expectation about our performance. There is a higher degree of regulation here, as well. City laws and codes are an extra burden on top of the heavy federal and state regulations. There are more unions in New York, and everything is more expensive. Because of the high expense and shortage of housing, recruitment of staff, particularly residents and nurses, is very difficult. If your hospital cannot provide subsidized housing for your nurses, then it's not competitive. On the positive side, New York does provide a certain excitement and vitality to the institution. That and the added pressure do push the institution and its people to higher levels of performance.

What is different about being the administrator of a not-for-profit hospital?
The voluntary, not-for-profit hospital is different from the other two forms of hospital organization in this country: government institutions and for-profit hospitals. The differences fall into two basic categories: first, the product or services being offered; and second, the management styles and attitudes.

The product is different in that the government hospitals are aimed at providing services to specific groups, usually the poor, the mentally ill, or veterans of the armed services. The for-profit institutions tend to provide those services from which they can make a profit. They, therefore, do not get involved in the expensive or complex patient care programs. The nonprofit hospitals, on the other hand, fill the need that the other two groups do not. They remain community-oriented for the populations not served by the public hospitals and at the same time must provide those services not considered by the profit sector for the general population. We have a commitment to provide full services to the entire community.

In terms of management styles, I think the not-for-profit hospital has less bureaucracy than the public sector and more accountability to the community than the for-profit group. The administrator in a profit-making hospital is less the master of his own ship, especially in the large hospital chains that have developed recently. This is because either the board or the central corporate office demands greater accountability and probably imposes certain standards for profit that limit options. The government hospitals tend to have a more public service attitude about management; the tax levy still provides a bail out for most government hospitals, and that removes a great deal of the pressure for good management from the administrative staff. I believe the expectations of our patients and medical staffs in the voluntary sector are probably the highest of the three groups. We probably have more flexibility in management, which I believe results in healthier and more reliable institutions. We are definitely more community-oriented than the for-profit sector, and, because of the reimbursement systems employed for the nonprofit hospitals, we have pressure not found in the government hospitals for good management.

How do you see the roles, tasks, and activities of hospital administrators changing over the next ten years?

The fifties and sixties represented a great growth period for the hospital industry. Administrators like to think of that period as the golden era. The seventies saw heavy regulation enter the scene and, in New York State, a severe cutback of dollars available for health care. This was a very serious business, and hospitals retrenched during that decade. The eighties in New York will probably be more of a steady state, with a continuation of the retrenching efforts within the industry outside New York. There will probably be a great deal of emphasis on cost containment as funds become scarcer and the industry is forced to come to grips with this. Other possibilities may emerge, such as the growth of HMOs. If President Reagan's competition ideas are implemented, you may see major changes, but these ideas are still not fully developed and to work require a great deal of legislative change. I don't think they will amount to as much as their proponents are hoping for.

At University Hospital I would like to see us get involved in more entrepreneurial activities. This may be the only way that we can grow. We face competition from the for-profit organizations, and current reimbursement mechanisms do not provide for adequate capital formation. We rely, therefore, on borrowing and philanthropy. It is exceedingly difficult to make big programmatic changes. Areas where I believe there is good opportunity include outpatient diagnostic services. Surpluses generated in these areas will facilitate other programmatic changes.

Program definition and matching resources to these programs are activities that will become more important in the next ten years. Hospitals are increasingly being put into groups of "like" institutions by the third-party payers. You will be forced to pay a penalty if you are not similar enough to the group in which you are classified. Hospitals will have to figure out where they are and where they want to be going. At University Hospital, we are starting to educate our trustees so they can be more supportive in this effort. If institutions are going to survive through the eighties, they will have to deal directly with the issues of mission, program size, program scope. A hospital cannot afford to be all things to all people. As a result, regionalization may become more of a reality during the eighties.

Administratively, we must organize so that our institutions can be responsive on fairly short notice to changes that are either advantageous to the institution or imposed on us from without. Management of change in the environment, as well as within the institution, will be a major challenge for the administrators in the eighties.

XI
From an Administrator's Files

It is about a search, too, for daily meaning as well as daily bread,
for recognition as well as cash, for astonishment rather than torpor;
in short for a sort of life rather than a Monday through Friday sort
of dying.

Studs Terkel

The items in this chapter are based on documents collected by a hospital administrator between December 1977 and March 1979. They have been edited to conceal the identities of the persons involved. I include them to provide a better and more direct idea of the job of the health services manager. Rather than being representative of what the manager does, these documents were selected to illustrate problem areas in one manager's job.

The following is a list of the documents contained in this chapter.

Item 1:   Letter from Community Hospital chief executive officer (CEO) to executive director of Southern Health Systems Agency about composition of hospital board of trustees. This letter was shared with the board chairman and never sent to the Health Systems Agency.

Item 2:   Letter from CEO Community Hospital to mayor of East City about city payment for indigent care. This letter was never responded to by the mayor. The CEO met with the mayor subsequently; the mayor "could do nothing" but was "supportive" of the hospital.

Item 3:   Letter from Community Hospital CEO to chief of police of East City about auto fatalities. This letter was never responded to by the chief of police; one of his assistants called and said that they were "concerned" about the problem.

Item 4:   Letter from Community Hospital CEO to chairman of the board of First Bank of East City about honoring contributions pledge. This letter was never responded to.

Item 5:   Letter from the chairman of radiology to Community Hospital CEO complaining about the CEO's behavior at a medical executive committee meeting.

Item 6:   Response of CEO to letter from chairman of radiology.

Item 7:   Letter from executive director of Southern Professional Standards Review Organization to Community Hospital CEO regarding medical care evaluation.

Item 8:   Letter from patient's father to president of Lexo Cement: copy to Community Hospital CEO, regarding hospital costs.

Item 9:   Response from Community Hospital CEO to letter from patient's father.

Item 10:   Minutes of the evaluation committee of the board of trustees meeting concerning board self-evaluation.

Item 11:   Board policy statements.

Item 12:   Committee objectives—1978.

Item 13:   Criteria and script questions from director of personnel for recruiting a new director of nursing at Community Hospital. The new director was chosen, in part, on the basis of candidates' answers to these questions.

Item 14:   A proposal from the controller to the CEO regarding medical staff contributions. This proposal was never shared with the medical staff or the board of trustees.

Item 15:   A proposal from the Community Hospital CEO to the president of the medical staff for a new medical reappointment worksheet. The proposal was rejected by the president of the medical staff; the existing form was retained.

Item 16:   Complaint from the chairman of pediatrics to Community Hospital CEO regarding special care nursery staff. The nursery was never closed.

Item 17:   Response from Community Hospital CEO to the chairman of pediatrics' complaint.

Item 18:   Memo from the head of the department of laboratories to Community Hospital CEO regarding physician authority, staffing, and cost in the department. Nothing was done in response to this memo.

Item 19:   Memo from executive secretary to Community Hospital CEO regarding patient complaint about quality of care. The executive secretary called the patient's mother and told her what action the hospital had taken, as indicated in Item 20.

Item 20:   Letter from the chairman of emergency services to Community Hospital CEO regarding patient complaint.

Item 1: Letter from Community Hospital CEO to Executive Director of Southern Health Systems Agency

October 24, 1978

Mr. Clement Full
Executive Director, Southern Region
Health Systems Agency
East State

Dear Mr. Full,

Our hospital Board of Trustees disagrees with the Southern Region Health Systems Agency's proposed project review guidelines (see attachment) for the following reasons:

1. Your own board has been regarded by many, including the HSA's own consultant, as ineffective because of its size and the difficulty in attracting effective members who meet a large number of demographic criteria.

2. There is little, if any, evidence in scientific journals proving that "acceptability" and "accessibility" of services is "problematic" in the cases where staff and policymaking bodies are not "representative" of the target population. The results I am familiar with indicate the opposite—namely, that patients want effective health services, that they see little need for representation of minorities on boards, nor do they think this will result in more effective health care. This is certainly patently obvious with respect to referral services such as CAT scanning or certain cancer treatment. For example, Joseph L. Falkson in his "An Evaluation of Alternative Modes of Citizen Participation in Urban Bureaucracy" summarizes on p. 162:

> Neither satisfaction with health services, nor long-term utilization rates were responsive to participatory initiatives. In fact, utilization rates were most responsive to better organized and financed bureaucracy-controlled (less participatory) health centers than to the more flexible and dynamic storefront program.

Similar results were found by J.J. Schwartz in his "Medical Plans and Health Care," on consumer participation in prepaid group practice plan governance.

3. Implementation will be difficult concerning changing the mix of government boards in time to meet planned submission schedules for certain needed project requests.

Our hospital currently has representation of racial and linguistic minorities and women (not the handicapped: Is anyone suggesting the mentally retarded?) on our governing board. In appropriately caring for patients in our catchment area, we have made significant attempts to increase employment of people with such characteristics, with some success.

The HSA should indicate to provider organizations how the HSA intends to use the proposed guidelines. There is nothing wrong with asking the indicated questions, but surely all projects should not be refused, for example, if the community is 58% female and there are only 10% females on the board, while there are 70% females on the staff and only 35% female supervisors.

Sincerely,

Victor Alan
Chief Executive Officer

VA/pg

*Amendments to Review Criteria**

1. Does the applicant's or program's staff reflect the target population it proposes to serve in the staff's composition?
2. Does the applicant have a governing body and/or advisory board(s)? Does the composition of the board(s) reflect the community and/or target area the applicant intends to serve? What mechanisms, established or envisioned, exist to assure effective participation of community representatives in the direction of broad policy decisions of the organization?

---

*Approved by the Southern Health Systems Agency's executive committee, June 21, 1979

Item 2: Letter from Community Hospital CEO to Mayor of East City

December 19, 1977

Mayor John Ricardo
East City

Dear Mayor Ricardo:

As you are aware, Community Hospital, East City's only general hospital, offers a wide range of needed services to all members of the East City community. The cost of providing these needed services has risen sharply since 1967, while the hospital has received from East City since 1967 the same annual appropriation of $33,000 per year. This amount is supposed to cover the cost of caring for the city's low-income families who have no insurance. The cost per day to care for indigent patients has risen from $46.51 in 1967 to $174.49 for the budget year 1978.

As you can see, the cost of services has risen over 350%; the amount of the appropriation has remained constant. It is important to recognize that the initial appropriation was insufficient to pay the hospital for the cost of providing care to East City's indigents. We estimate the cost of 1979 to be about $340,000 per year. As you know, Medicare, Medicaid, and Blue Cross do not reimburse the hospital for any free care provided to East City's indigents. Community Hospital is asking your support to present to the city council a budget for increasing the hospital appropriation, to more adequately cover our costs.

We thank you for your consideration in this matter and anxiously await a positive response. I would be happy to discuss this matter further with you at your earliest convenience. In any event, I look forward to meeting you and wish to learn of your ideas concerning improving hospital services.

Sincerely,

Victor Alan
Chief Executive Officer

VA/nd

bcc: Controller
    Board Chairman

Item 3: Letter from Community Hospital CEO to Chief of Police of East City

October 5, 1978

Timothy Rowland
Chief of Police
East City

Dear Chief Rowland:

The recent and tragic death of 12-year-old Timmy Lucas, who was hit by a car on Lakesville Bridge Road, rekindles my deep concern with appropriate motor vehicle safety in East City. East City and Varek County's death rates from motor vehicle accidents are the worst in the state, according to the local Health Systems Agency; in fact, they are twice the state average.

Can you share with me any information for the last three years regarding where fatalities and serious accidents take place, at what times of the day, how often, and the ages of those involved? Also, what is the police department doing to lower those rates of motor vehicle deaths and serious injuries?

I recognize that motor vehicle safety is a complicated and difficult problem. It is, however, I am convinced, one of the most serious health problems in East City. Please let me know of any way I or our hospital staff can help you in this effort.

Sincerely,

Victor Alan
Chief Executive Officer

VA/nd

Item 4: Letter from Community Hospital CEO to Chairman of the Board of First Bank of East City

December 11, 1978

Mr. George Ricarelli
Chairman
First Bank of East City

Dear Mr. Ricarelli,

It has recently been called to my attention that Community Hospital has not received any payments from the First Bank of East City toward their modernization fund pledge of $30,000. This pledge was to be used to establish the main reception area, located on the ground floor of the new west wing of our hospital. Several letters to your bank have gone un-answered, and recent remarks allow me to believe that some degree of misunderstanding exists. Might we visit to resolve this matter?

Our new west wing is nearing completion and, correlatively, construction payments must be made. The uncertain status of a pledge of this magnitude greatly concerns me, and I therefore respectfully request your personal attention to the resolution of this situation.

In the interest of providing you with some background information, I have attached a copy of a newspaper clipping from the August 1, 1977, edition of the *East City Daily Sentinel* announcing the intended contribution. Also, other financial institutions have made the following pledges to this most recent and important fund-raising campaign.

First Bank of East City	$30,000
National Savings & Loan	25,000
State Bank	15,000
Richmond National Bank	6,000
First National Bank of Clark	6,000
Silver Bank	3,000
Carl's Savings & Loan	3,000
Fourth Federal Savings & Loan	1,500

Thanking you in advance for your anticipated cooperation, and hoping to hear from you in the very near future, I am

Very truly yours,

Samuel Brocetti
Community Hospital Board of
Trustees

bcc: Chief Executive Officer
Chairman, Finance Committee
Controller

Item 5: Letter from the Chairman of Radiology to Community Hospital CEO

September 15, 1979

Mr. Victor Alan
Chief Executive Officer
Community Hospital

Dear Mr. Alan,

I am writing to you to convey to you in writing my feelings with respect to the medical executive committee meeting on Monday, September 11, 1978.

As you are aware, one of the topics on the agenda for discussion that evening by the medical board members was medical services. It was felt by several department chairmen who sit on the medical executive committee that we would profit from a discussion of medical services at Community Hospital and the status of obtaining needed medical equipment to provide these services.

You heard the *chairman of radiology* discuss the fact that the Hospital has had to control the planned radiology capital budget for 1978 because of the need to replace some equipment on an emergency basis. I then repeated my view, so that medical board members could be informed of it, that in a department with such high capital costs it is imperative that planned acquisition and replacement of equipment be allowed to proceed without further cancellation. We cannot budget to replace equipment over a period of 15 years, for instance, when the equipment has a life expectancy of only 8 years, on average. I felt that the entire medical board must recognize this unfortunate drain on the total medical capital budget, which will persist year after year. Interdepartment cooperation will become increasingly necessary to insure that the radiology capital budget does not act to the detriment of the other departments' budgets. If the monies are not provided, the department will in a few years suddenly be presented with very severe function problems, and the Hospital, in turn, will be faced with very large capital expenditures. I also felt that we should be rapidly advancing into areas of diagnosis which are of benefit to our patients and which allow us to remain competitive with surrounding hospitals that are developing these capabilities.

You heard the *chairman of medicine* voice his concerns that the Hospital was not providing some services which he felt it should and which are generally becoming available in progressive surrounding facilities. He is referring, in part, to cardiac stress testing associated with nuclear medicine cardiovascular capability. The comments would, however, hold equally well for other areas.

You heard the *chairman of surgery* comment on the technically poor quality of the angiograms which can be provided at Community Hospital because of our inferior equipment and lack of a dedicated angiographic system. He compared them to the quality of the studies that are being generated by Miller Hospital, which he feels are vastly superior. This impacts significantly on his decisions as to appropriate types of vascular surgery for his patients. In addition, we are currently capable of performing no angiographic studies of any kind. This was, I think, dramatically illustrated when, during our meeting, he received word that a patient had been transported from Miller to Community for arteriography and, hopefully, vascular surgery for gangrene of the foot, only to have to send the patient back to Miller for the appropriate arteriographic studies so that a decision could be made as to whether or not to operate at Community. He generally commented on the fact that it was the responsibility of the medical board—and, indeed, the entire hospital—to strive to provide top quality services in spite of those factors operating against the development of these services.

You heard the *chairman of anesthesiology* discuss the fact that he was saddled with some anesthetic equipment which is of such a state he deemed it a danger to patients. You also heard him mention the fact that there was no ongoing service maintenance or quality control testing done on this type of equipment in his department by the Hospital.

You heard a member of the *division of gastroenterology* report on the recent decrease in service which can be provided by the nuclear medicine section because of administrative decisions which prohibit section employees from collecting overtime. This is in spite of the fact that we currently are performing, on average, twice as many studies as nearby hospitals of comparable size with only one-half the equipment and too few technologists. He mentioned that he has had to refer patients from Community to Richmond for nuclear medicine scans. It has been taking up to a week for the nuclear medicine section to complete some of the studies because of the heavy demand and limited capability relative to progressive institutions of this size.

You heard discussion that the *staff* had not even been able to obtain cheap Doppler type equipment for the evaluation of patients with actual or impending strokes.

The *chairman of urology* has informed me that the department has been unable to obtain some needed equipment and that this has resulted in major surgical procedures being performed on members of our community when otherwise relatively minor procedures would have sufficed.

In summary, multiple concerns were expressed, and, since some of the department chairmen were unaware of the other departments' difficulties, I feel that the result of the meeting was quite informative and productive.

As mentioned above, these discussions were for the information and benefit of the medical executive committee physicians and were not a report or proposal, either formal or informal, to the administration or trustees. The medical board members are charged by the hospital trustees with the professional, medical operation of this hospital, and discussions of this type are, obviously, necessary and proper. As the chief executive officer, you sit as a welcome and invited guest at these meetings of the medical executive committee, and your comment was naturally anticipated.

I was disappointed in that your response seemed to be somewhat defensive, and I feel that you assumed the posture that we were in an advisory relationship. I feel that several of your statements at this point were unfortunate.

Your comment that, since so many things were necessary, personnel reductions would be required in those departments where the number of personnel were excessive and the volume of work was decreasing was not misunderstood by me. I consider it was intended as a veiled threat to members of the medical executive committee who had discussed topics that you perhaps did not wish to have discussed. I would remind you that the MEC meetings are our meetings and are designed for exactly this type of discussion. I repeat, your statements were not misunderstood by me, since you had couched similar statements in exactly the same phraseology during our recent trip to Clark Memorial Hospital for meetings concerning the CAT scanner. I immediately repeated for your edification that the work load in the radiology department through the end of August, 1978, when compared with the previous year, was decreased by approximately one and one-half percent. A great portion of this slight change results from anticipated seasonal fluctuations, along with recent decreases in hospital admissions. I do not feel that the department statistics as reflected in the trustees' financial report of July, 1978, warrant this type of statement.

I also feel that the timing of this type of statement was inappropriate, since we were in no way attempting to negotiate or work out solutions with the administration at that particular meeting.

Your statement that $600,000, which would ordinarily be spent towards the acquisition of a CAT scanner, might have to be utilized to address some of the other needs expressed by the board members puzzled me, since I do not think that reflects the current wishes of the medical staff or the board of trustees.

Your comment that the hospital had spent $343,000 during the past year on the radiology department was, I feel, somewhat misleading in that a major portion of this expense is not reflected in the figures I have available and must somehow refer in large part to items funded under the expansion-bond program. In any event, the administration has thus far been unable to inform me exactly which items are included under various financing arrangements. I should very much like to have that information. I would also appreciate being informed of the details as to why the proposed radiology expansion project has thus far not been approved by the state, as you mentioned in your administrator's report.

Finally, your statement that we were indirectly implying that the trustees were not doing their job was most ill-advised, since you had previously been specifically advised by several speakers that we recognize the financial pressures upon the Hospital and were not implying anything about the lay board. The implications were, rather, that the medical board members may have been deficient in the past in not jointly discussing needs between departments. To this end, I suggested establishing a sub-committee to insure that the major medical chairmen are aware of not only their own needs but the needs of the other departments so that a reasonable balance of budgetary priorities can be accomplished. This would also result in, in the future, more comprehensive, thought-out requests being submitted by the medical staff for trustee consideration. There is also some feeling, which I have heard, that perhaps the medical representatives to the board of trustees have not been adequately reflecting the feelings of the department chairmen with respect to the development of medical services; again, we probably have to improve our own function in this respect and insure that we maintain better communication with our own representatives. In no case, and you were specifically told this, was an implication being made about the trustees; for you to attempt to imply this at the end of your statements concerns me greatly. The medical board is not trying to confront the trustees in any manner.

In summarizing, I can only say that you were privy to discussions occurring between the physician members of the medical executive committee and are certainly welcome to continue doing this. I feel that some of your statements were ill-advised and of an intimidating nature, and I should hate to see the situation arise where medical executive committee members do not feel comfortable in discussing matters at their meetings that are their responsibility because of your presence. If this occurs, there will have been a very serious breakdown in communications between the administration and the medical staff, and the current trustees and medical staff have worked too long and too hard over these past several years to have this occur.

Hoping that we can work progressively together in the future, I remain

                                   Sincerely,

                                   Alexander Greenspan, M.D.
                                   Chairman of Radiology

AG/ll

cc: Board of Trustees
    Medical Executive Committee

P.S. I have learned that the morning following the medical board meeting you notified the department of anesthesiology that they would be obtaining some additional, badly needed equipment. I feel this again points out the positive nature of these types of discussions.

Item 6: Response of CEO to Letter from Chairman of Radiology

September 22, 1978

Alexander Greenspan, M.D.
Chief, Department of Radiology
Community Hospital

Dear Alex,

Your letter of September 15 contains serious inaccuracies and misstatements. They are as follows:

—I stated that capital equipment must be considered within the content of overall departmental expenditures, and, in departments where there have been volume decreases, this must be taken into consideration. This applies to all departments and was no "veiled threat" to your department.

—I stated that acquiring a CAT scanner would have to be considered in relation to other hospital capital equipment needs. The medical staff and the board of trustees should express their thoughts in this matter, and I ask them to do so by all means.

—One of the physicians present at the MEC meeting said it was the board's job to raise the money necessary to buy new equipment. I was responding to his comment by saying that I thought that the trustees and the medical staff had done an excellent job in raising money for capital projects and must continue to do so.

—The anesthesia equipment you mention in your postscript had already been approved for purchase in 1978 prior to the MEC meeting.

I share your concerns and those of the MEC about appropriate and timely equipping of our hospital. (Your requests pertaining to radiology purchasing and state approval will be answered under separate cover.) A meeting with the finance committee to discuss capital equipment needs, with Dr. Black, Dr. Blue, and yourself (Dr. Handley is unable to attend), has been set for Tuesday, October 17, at 4:15 p.m.

I feel that in no way were my statements to the medical executive committee "ill-advised or of an intimidating nature." I certainly did not mean them to be so. Several physicians apologized to me afterwards for the rudeness shown me during the meeting, as I was not even allowed to speak without frequently being interrupted.

I pledge to work progressively together with you and the medical executive committee as you urge in your letter.

Sincerely,

Victor Alan
Chief Executive Officer

VA/nd

cc: Joseph Brocetti
    President of the Board of Trustees

Lisle Kent
President of the Medical Staff

Item 7: Letter from Executive Director of Southern Professional Standards Review Organization to Community Hospital CEO

March 28, 1979

Victor Alan
Administrator
Community Hospital

Dear Mr. Alan,

On March 14th our organization conducted a quarterly monitoring survey at your hospital. The survey included a review of both the concurrent review and the medical care evaluation activities. The team members who surveyed your concurrent review program noted that both the admission certification and the discharge planning portions of the program were timely and effective. Considerable improvement was noted in the continued stay review activities, and an increase in physician participation and documentation was evident. The most serious problem detected in the continued stay review portion of your program is that your physician advisors continue to review questionable cases at a time later than they should be reviewed. A more detailed summary of the concurrent review monitor is attached.

Pertaining to the medical care evaluation portion of your program, the team noted that some improvement is needed in order for you to have a first-rate medical care evaluation study program. Your committee members need assistance in developing criteria and in addressing variation analysis. In addition, the audit plan, which currently is in final draft form, should be submitted to us at the earliest practical date. One final recommendation would be that the audit committee develop a dialogue with the utilization review committee, and vice versa, in order to provide for an ongoing exchange of information. A copy of the survey recommendations for your MCE program is attached.

As a result of the monitoring survey, your hospital will continue in a delegated status. Your program meets the PSRO program requirements, and I feel certain that it will continue to improve with increased physician interest and expertise. May I take this opportunity to thank you and your staff for the hospitality which you extended to the team members?

Sincerely yours,

Philip A. Mercado
Executive Director

PAM/bb
Enclosure

Item 8: Memo from Patient's Father to President of Lexo Cement: copy to Community Hospital CEO

Lexo Cement Corporation
Interoffice Memorandum

TO: Stephen Volare   Office: Flaret
FROM: M.B. Collar   Office: Richmond
SUBJECT: Enclosed Hospital Billing   Date: March 2, 1979

Dear Stephen:

I received this statement for a hospital stay and surgery for my son.

My son entered the hospital around 7:00 p.m. 2/13/79. He spent that night and the next day in the hall until he went to surgery at approximately 6:00 p.m. 2/14/79. He, incidentally, had no meals from the time he entered until surgery. Following surgery, he was returned to Room 236, a semi-private room, and remained there until 10:30 a.m. 2/15/79, at which time I brought him home.

I called the hospital to protest the billing, and in particular the room charge, and was informed that it was customary to charge semi-private rates even to sleep in the hall. That is an outrage!

I hope there is something our carrier can do to dispute this billing. It is no wonder that our premiums are so high.

MBC

Attachment

Copy to: Community Hospital
         Attn: Hospital Administrator

Community Hospital

Slept in hall and remained
in hall until surgery 2/14
@ 6 p.m. Returned to room
9:00 p.m. Discharged 10:30
a.m. 2/15.

When referring to this account
please use admission no.

1-06277-7	02/15/79
Admission No.	Discharge Date

Regular   02/20/79   Page 1

Collar, Horace   Age 17   Phy 231   01

Date	Ref. No.	Desc. Code	Service Description	Quant.	Price
			Date of Admission 02/13/79		
		*** 01	Room & Board		
2/13		299	Semi-Private at 125.00 per	1	125.00
2/14		206	Semi-Private at 125.00 day	1	125.00
			Area Total ***	2	250.00
		*** 16	Laboratory-Hematology		
2/14	060	0801-7	CBC B628		8.40
			Area Total ***		8.40
		*** 26	Laboratory-Urinalysis		
	061	2102-7	Routine Analysis B934		5.25
			Area Total ***		5.25
		*** 36	X ray		
2/15	200	3130-6	Hand A261		22.00
2/15	200	6130-3	Port. X-ray Exam		16.00
			Bedside or O.R.		
			Area Total ***		38.00
		*** 50	Pharmacy		
2/16	245	0002-1	Medication	3	1.35
2/16	245	0003-9	Medication	3	7.20
2/16	245	1100-2	Medication		8.85
2/16	245	1100-2	Medication	2	17.70
2/16	245	9999-9	Above Chgs Surgery &		
			Floor Drugs		N/C
2/17	311	0002-1	Medication		.45
2/17	311	0003-9	Medication	3	7.20
2/17	311	1100-2	Medication	10	88.50
			Area Total ***		131.25

		*** 79	Operating Room		
2/15	212	0001-2	Operating Room	10	600.00
2/15	212	1000-3	General Supplies		100.00
			Area Total ***		700.00
		*** 80	Central Supply		
2/16	194	9999-6	Basin Set		6.00
2/16	283	0000-2	Central Sterile Supplies		65.00
			Area Total ***		71.00

Community Hospital

When referring to this account,
please use admissions no.

Malcolm Collar	1-06277-7	02-15-79
	Admissions No.	Discharge Date

Regular	02/20/79	Page 2

Collar, Horace   Age 17   Phy 231   01

Date	Ref. No.	Desc. Code	Service Description	Quan.	Price
		*** 82	I.V. Solutions	4	38.00
	212	0001-6	I.V. Solutions		
2/15	212	0010-7	Standard Administration Kit		4.75
2/15	212	0250-9	Cannulla, Medicut		4.75
2/16	242	0000-8	General		2.50
2/16	242	0001-6	I.V. Solutions		9.50
2/17	310	0000-8	General		2.50
2/17	310	0001-6	I.V. Solutions	5	47.50
			Area Total ***		109.50
		*** 92	Telephone		
2/15	194	0001-5	Regular		1.00
			Area Total ***		1.00
			Total Charges		*** 1,314.00
		*** 99	Payments		1.00
2/15	250916	00	Patient Payment		1.00
			Area Total***		
			Balance Due		1,313.40
			2/23/79 BC NJ allow		1,313.40
					0.00

Item 9: Response from Community Hospital CEO to Letter from Patient's Father

March 13, 1979

Mr. Malcolm Collar

Dear Mr. Collar,

In response to the interoffice memo of March 2, a copy of which you sent me, the hospital costs allocable to the occasional patient who must be temporarily accommodated in the hall are not significantly different than for the patient hospitalized in a semi-private room—such costs include nursing care, utilities, housekeeping, and so forth. High quality hospital care is expensive. Premiums would be even higher if excess hospital capacity were built and licensed so that no one would ever have to be cared for in the hall.

It is theoretically possible to construct a charging system so that patients would be charged only for services that they use, such as meals actually eaten. The costs of administering such a system (with the large number of different governmental and third-party payer requirements related to reimbursement which all hospitals face) would probably result in higher costs to all patients. The cost of developing such a system would be inordinate for our hospital. In any event, the new system would only result in charging some patients more and other patients less for hospital costs, which would remain the same, in providing care to all our patients.

I do understand your concern for high health insurance premium costs. You should know, however, that Community Hospital is a relatively low-cost hospital in a state where hospital costs are significantly lower than those of hospitals in the rest of the United States. Such lower costs should be reflected in your company's health insurance premiums as a state firm purchasing Blue Cross.

I hope I have answered the questions raised by the copy of the letter you sent me and would be happy to discuss this further with you, if you like.

Sincerely,

Victor Alan
Chief Executive Officer

VA/nd
cc: S. Volare
   J. Brocetti
   President, Community Hospital Board of Trustees

Item 10: Minutes of the Evaluation Committee of the Board of Trustees Meeting, July 21, 1978

Present: Ms. Brown, Mr. Strong, Mr. Brocetti, Dr. Ringo, Mr. Alan

The committee reviewed the results of the self-evaluation forms completed by board members. Some highlights:

A. Key Responsibilities—Very Important
Evaluating the CEO (18)
Setting Hospital Goals and Policies (17)
Long-Range Planning (16)
Reviewing Annual Budget (16)

B. Very Effective Areas for the Board
Reviewing Medical Staff Performance (6)
Raising Funds (5)
Reviewing Annual Budget (5)

C. Not Very Effective Areas for the Board
Reviewing Medical Staff Performance (5)
Communicating with Regulators and Public Officials (5)
Building Community Ties (5)

D. Some Sample Suggestions
   1. Do not read committee minutes, cover only action items.
   2. Improve trustee orientation.
   3. Determine areas of board weakness and recruit selectively to fill same.
   4. Organize monthly meetings better.
   5. Inform total board of problems that involve both physicians and the hospital.
   6. Give board members more choice in committee assignments.
   7. Do not automatically reelect present board members.
   8. Schedule trustee tours through various departments.
   9. Reduce size of the board to 15.
   10. Executive committee should be smaller, used more frequently.

It was suggested that attendance be recorded at all committee meetings, as with general board meetings, with results tabulated and prepared for the president of the board.

It was recommended that the attached form regarding *Appraising the Activity of Peers* be filled out by board members in October. Each board member will fill in 17 sheets on each other board member and will give them to Mr. Brocetti, who will tabulate. There will be no identification of who filled the sheets out. Each board member will then receive a summary of his own ratings and comments about his performance from Mr. Brocetti. The purpose of peer evaluation is as follows: (1) to help individual trustees perform better; (2) to aid in reelection decisions; (3) to increase accountability of board members to each other and the board.

The committee recommended a one-day education seminar for trustees to be held during the fall of the year.

The committee approved conceptually of an outside evaluation of the nursing department to upgrade performance.

At the next meeting, to be held on September 8, 1978, evaluation of the CEO will be discussed further.

Respectfully submitted,

Victor Alan
Chief Executive Officer

VA/nd

Item 11: Community Hospital Board Policy Statements

Term of Office	Term of each member be extended to five years.	10/26/66
Signing of Documents	Treasurer shall be allowed to sign documents in the absence of the secretary.	6/26/68
Consecutive Years of Service	No trustee shall serve for more than ten consecutive years. Eligible for election again after one year off the board.	11/27/68
Signature Required	One signature required on all accounts payable checks.	3/31/70
Safety Deposit Box	A member of the board and the administrator be present at all times the safety deposit box is opened.	3/28/72
No Smoking	Sales of cigarettes discontinued in the hospital.	7/26/76
Capital Expenditures	Finance committee up to $5,000 and CEO up to $3,000 without board approval.	2/28/77
Malpractice	The board will rule on all cases to be settled, upon recommendations from our lawyer. Policy guidelines to be established.	6/27/77
Abortion	Hospital cannot forbid performing of abortions, per court decision.	6/27/77
Discounts	Discontinue discounts for physicians, clergy, and trustees immediately, except as covered in the employee handbook.	8/29/77
Solicitation	No employee may solicit or distribute materials during working time in working areas.	10/31/77
Foundation	A foundation to be established with monies	10/31/77

	earmarked for Community Hospital's specific needs.	
Collections	Care shall be provided when urgently needed by patients, but every appropriate attempt shall be made to collect monies due the hospital.	11/28/77
Quality Assurance	Medical department heads to set goals and report annually on performance.	1/30/78
Patient's Bill of Rights	Board of trustees adopted Patient's Bill of Rights. (This bill will become part of Community Hospital's patient booklet.)	2/27/78
Minutes	Board minutes to be shared with medical executive committee.	2/27/78
Administrator Authority to Purchase or Lease Equipment	Administrator given authority to make the decision to purchase or lease equipment already approved for purchase costing $10,000 or less.	4/24/78
AHA Resolution	Board of trustees adopted AHA national voluntary cost-containment resolution.	4/24/78
Nepotism	Nepotism clause adopted by board of trustees. Policy does not affect those employees working prior to 5/1/78.	5/22/78
Philosophy of Service	Philosophy of service policy adopted by board of trustees.	10/30/78
Policy on Conflict of Interest	A policy on conflict of interest and disclosure statement for board members and key managers adopted by the board of trustees.	11/27/78

Item 12: Committee Objectives—1978

General
1. The president will be an ex officio member of all committees, *with* the right to vote.
2. All committee members, including department heads and community representatives, shall have the right to vote.
3. The chief executive officer will have the right to vote on all committees to which the president has appointed him. The chief executive officer or his assistant will be ex officio members of all other committees, *without* the right to vote.
4. Committee chairmen will nominate, receive board approval, and appoint at least one community representative to the following committees: purchasing and finance, building and grounds, personnel, annual dinner-dance, fund-raising, foundation, and planning.
5. In addition to the committee responsibilities indicated in the bylaws, the following specific committee objectives will be addressed in 1978.

Executive
1. Shall convene as requested by the president to address special hospital matters and advise resolution of said matters.

Purchasing and Finance
1. Develop cash forecasts and contingency plans to deal with cash shortfalls.
2. Attempt to make monthly report on hospital's financial position.
3. Explore and evaluate alternative revenue sources.
4. Establish targets or goals for days outstanding in accounts receivable and accounts payable.
5. Develop and implement an appropriate capital budgeting process.
6. Develop variable budgeting program relating to volume changes for 1979.
7. Develop an effective materials management program.

Joint Conference
1. Improve communications among board, administration, and medical staff.
2. Discuss obstacles to and opportunities for the elimination of low-quality care.
3. Discuss the financial position of the hospital and methods of improving same.
4. Discuss methods used and progress made in recruiting new physicians to the East City Community.

Building and Grounds
1. Monitor the development of each year's capital budget for all expenditures related to plant, property, and equipment.
2. Monitor the development, implementation, and continual evaluation of a plan which assures that all physical facilities meet necessary requirements for full accreditation by the proper authorities.
3. Monitor the development, implementation, and continual evaluation of a program for regular, routine, and preventive maintenance of plant, property, and equipment.
4. Monitor the development, implementation, and continual evaluation of a program which assesses, and reduces when appropriate, the total energy consumption of the hospital.
5. Regularly review the policies, procedures, job descriptions, and so on that relate to personnel in the plant operations department, to insure that the department is adequately and properly staffed to carry out the objectives of this committee at the lowest possible expense.
6. Monitor the new expansion project to insure completion on schedule and within budget.
7. Provide input to the purchasing and finance committee in the development of a land acquisition policy.
8. Evaluate all parking considerations and requirements, and develop and implement a program to meet those requirements.
9. Develop a plan for the utilization of the space vacated by the relocation into the new expansion facilities.

Annual Dinner-Dance
1. Strive for highest quality event.
2. Increase community involvement, especially by doctors' wives, and thereby improve public relations.
3. Obtain greater newspaper coverage of actual event.
4. Increase profit.
5. Evaluate other potential locations.
6. Update mailing list.
7. Obtain appointment of hospital employee to be responsible for details and coordination with chairman.

Fund Raising
1. Follow last fund-raising campaign to insure that maximum pledge dollars are collected.
2. Identify, initiate, and establish at least one additional method of securing funds for hospital in 1978.
3. Increase funds raised.
4. Identify fund-raising "master plan".

Nominating
1. Define areas of expertise required for well-balanced board and identify areas of expertise that are lacking on present board.
2. Establish list of potential trustees. Supply this list to committee chairmen and obtain candidate appointment to committees. Evaluate interest and performance.
3. Nominate three (3) new trustees by December 1, 1978.

Planning
1. Reorganize committee according to most recent consultant's recommendations.
2. Establish, assign priority to, and update hospital goals on regular basis.
3. Organize committees for implementation in areas of long-term care, physical medicine, health education, same-day surgery, alcoholism, and joint planning.
4. Develop one new shared program or expand significantly an existing shared program with Russell and Regis hospitals.

Personnel
1. Implement annual evaluation program for all employees.
2. Address impact of growing Spanish-speaking community on personnel policies.
3. Recommend wage and benefit increases for hospital employees in 1979.
4. Consider employee unionization and recommend preventive policy.
5. Identify methods of improving employee morale.

Evaluation
1. Establish a method of evaluating chief executive officer.
2. Establish a method of evaluating board of trustees.

Legal and Bylaws
1. Evaluate existing bylaws and make suggestions regarding needed changes.

Foundation
1. Establish foundation and maximize assets.

Item 13: Criteria and Script Questions for Recruiting a New Director of Nursing at Community Hospital

---

A. *Criteria for Position of Director of Nursing*
   1. Gifted teacher of nursing management and nursing service.
   2. Respected clinician.
   3. Adequate knowledge of quality assurance.
   4. Ability to recruit effectively for qualified R.N.s.
   5. Effective motivator of nurses.
   6. Effective negotiator with medical staff and administration.
   7. Experience in structuring nursing service and in scheduling and staffing.
   8. Commitment to patient care and experience with effective patient teaching programs.

B. *Qualifications*
   1. Master's degree preferred.
   2. Relevant experience in nursing management at general hospital of 250 beds or larger.
   3. Ability to communicate orally and in writing.
   4. Familiarity with budgeting and statistics.
   5. Congenial, warm personality.

C. *Salary*
   $25,000–$30,000

Script Questions for Final Candidates

Name:

Day: Date: Time:

Notes:

Questions:
   1. How would you more effectively recruit R.N.s? For evening and night shifts? For weekend coverage?
   2. What is the appropriate nursing administration organization for a 235-bed general hospital?
   3. How would you gain the confidence of the medical staff?
   4. What would be your main contribution to improving nursing service?

5. What role should the nursing department play in patient education?
6. What experience have you had in controlling nursing costs? What results have you achieved?
7. What are your ideas on effective in-service education?
8. What are your ideas on effective quality assurance programs?
9. Have you had any experience with unions or nurse organizing? How do you feel about this?
10. What have you achieved in your present job?
11. How do you improve nursing morale?
12. How is nursing service different in a hospital without a house staff? What kind of problems do you anticipate?
13. What are you looking for in the position you are seeking? Why do you think you will find it here?
14. What would be your strengths and weaknesses as a director of nursing?
15. What basic qualifications do you think are most important for a director of nursing?

Questions Asked by Candidate:

Summary Discussion:

Item 14: A Proposal for Planned Medical Staff Contributions

In order for a hospital to maintain a sustained equipment and facilities acquisition and replacement program in such an unfavorable economic climate as that which currently exists in the state, there must be intensive and long-term efforts to generate contributions from affiliated physicians and from the community.

A good contribution plan for physicians should incorporate some consideration of the equipment and facilities needed by the hospital to support their particular specialities. A very good plan was developed by the administration of West Mannix Hospital. This plan incorporates weighted specialty factors that are intended to make donations relate to facilities usage. This plan, when coupled with an increase of $200 in medical staff dues, would produce an annual contribution of approximately $78,000. This plan would supplant the current random method for soliciting medical staff donations and would result in annual contributions ranging from $200 to maximum of $3,523.

It would be the understanding of the Hospital that the proceeds of this plan would be used for the purchase of that medical equipment which the medical executive committee deems most desirable.

Volume and Intensity Portion of the Plan

All physicians who treat more than 25 cases per year are included in the formula.

Specialty Factors

Family Practice, Pediatrics	3.1
Internal Medicine	4.0
Proctology, Otorhinolaryngology, Oral Surgery	4.4
Obstetrics, Gynecology, Ophthalmology	4.8
Urology	5.3
General Surgery, Neurology	5.7
Orthopedics, Plastic Surgery	6.3

The estimated annual contribution from the specialty factor computations shown on Schedule I (attached) is $59,602.

Increase in Physician Dues

An additional $200 per year per physician would produce approximately $18,600 in additional contributions.

Schedule 1: Computation of Speciality Factor Contributions

Total Physicians	Specialists	Specialty Factors	x	Cases	=	Annual Specialty Donations
13	Family Practice, Pediatrics	3.1	x	2,848	=	$ 8,829
9	Internal Medicine	4.0	x	1,626	=	6,504
3	Oral Surgery, Otorhinolaryngology	4.4	x	158	=	695
7	Obstetrics, Gynecology, Ophthalmology	4.8	x	2,290	=	10,992
4	Urology	5.3	x	383	=	2,030
5	General Surgery, Neurology	5.7	x	1,762	=	10,043
3	Orthopedics, Plastic Surgery	6.3	x	619	=	3,900
__44__	Total Admitting					$ __42,993__
	Average per Physician = $977 (a)					
5	Radiology		x	$ 977	=	$ 4,885
3	Anesthesiology		x	977	=	2,931
3	Pathology		x	977	=	2,931
6	Emergency Room		x	977	=	__5,862__
17	Total Hospital-Based					$ __16,609__
__61__	TOTAL					$ __59,602__

(a) $42,993 ÷ 44 = $ 977

Item 15: Proposal from the Community Hospital CEO to the President of the Medical Staff for a New Medical Reappointment Worksheet

December 13, 1978

To: Lisle Kent, M.D.
President of the Medical Staff

From: Victor Alan
Chief Executive Officer

Re: Reappointment Worksheet

Attached are my suggestions for a revised form. I claim no expertise in this area.

To work properly, letters and statements need to be placed in each physician's personnel file concerning the following:

—Problems with audit or utilization review
—Attendance at meetings
—Complaints and incidents
—Physical examinations
—Malpractice judgments

Confidentiality of files needs to be established so that these are accessible only to the department chief and the appropriate physician.

VA/nd
Att.

cc: Joseph Brocetti
President, Board of Trustees

Community Hospital

Name___________________________ Date___________________________

Address_________________________ Phone__________________________

Worksheet for Reappointment

	Excellent	Satisfactory	Unsatisfactory
Professional Competence and Clinical Judgment	______	______	______
Ethics and Conduct	______	______	______
Attendance at Medical Staff Meetings	______	______	______
Participation on Medical Staff Committees	______	______	______
Compliance with Hospital and Medical Staff Bylaws, Rules, and Regulations	______	______	______
Cooperation with Hospital Personnel	______	______	______
Rapport with Other Physicians	______	______	______
General Attitude toward Patients, Hospital, and the Public	______	______	______
Physical and Mental Capabilities	______	______	______
Evidence of Continuous Learning in His or Her Field	______	______	______

Summary:

Comments:

Department Chairman Signature_____________________________ Date________

Attending Physician Signature______________________________ Date________

Application for Reappointment to the Medical Staff
Community Hospital

Name———————— Date————

Office Address———— Phone————

Home Address———— Phone————

NOTE ANY *CHANGES* IN FOLLOWING
  SINCE LAST APPOINTMENT:

Teaching Appointments — Date————

Postgraduate Education — Date————

Membership on Other

Hospital Staffs———— Date————

Specialty Board Qualified— Date————

Certified by American

Board of———————— Date————

or

Status in Board

Certification Process———— Date————

List on Back Separately Scientific Papers Given, Scientific Meetings and
  CME Sessions Attended.

Have Your Privileges at Any Hospital Ever Been Suspended, Revoked, or
  Not Renewed?

                                        Yes———— No————

Has Your License To Practice Medicine in Any Jurisdiction Ever Been
  Suspended or Revoked?

                                        Yes———— No————

Have You Ever Been Convicted of a Crime or Felony?

                                        Yes———— No————

Have You Ever Been Named in a Malpractice Suit (Past 5 Years)?

                                        Yes———— No————

Have You Ever Had Your Narcotics License Suspended or Revoked?

                                        Yes———— No————

IF YOUR ANSWER TO ANY OF THE ABOVE QUESTIONS WAS
  YES, EXPLAIN IN FULL ON SEPARATE SHEET.

Do You Have Malpractice Insurance?

  Name of Carrier———————— Amount of Coverage————

My Present Appointment and Service Is ————————————

I Am Applying for Same or as Follows ————————————

————————————   ————————————
        Date   Signature

Item 16: Complaint from the Chairman of Pediatrics to Community Hospital CEO Regarding Special Care Nursery Staff

January 8, 1979

To: Victor Alan

From: Benjamin Ringo

I was unable to page you on Sunday afternoon, January 7, for another visit to our intensive care nursery, where an excellent labor room nurse from the delivery room had been placed in charge! She, of course, has never had the six-week orientation essential to knowing how to care for an acutely ill neonate, just like the situation I showed you last week with the nurse who cooked a premature infant for several hours to produce fever and distress because she had no knowledge or experience in handling a sick neonate or premature infant.

The labor room nurse in the intensive care nursery had to monitor an early, distressed, premature breech who had been delivered with an Apgar of 5. Needless to say, she was terribly upset with this awesome responsibility. I tried to console her.

The problem I write about continues unabated. In fact, the nurse who cooked the premature infant two weeks ago was placed in charge again on at least two other nights after the above episode.

If you intend to allow this situation to continue, that is, having such poorly staffed backup for such a critical care area, I respectfully suggest that you close down the unit and not deceive East City's citizens about the quality of care offered 24 hours daily, seven days weekly, to a sick neonate here.

I do understand that you are having difficulty in recruiting a new director of nursing. I wonder if some qualified people are reluctant to apply for a position you said was being managed well three months ago and then overnight decided wasn't and told the present director to step down or leave; all this occurring moments after Mrs. Gluck was fired.

Because Phil Strong has phoned me on several occasions to inquire about things, I have taken the liberty of sending this memo to him also. Please do give these matters your prompt, personal attention.

cc: P. Strong, Vice-President of the Board

Item 17: Response from Community Hospital CEO to the Chairman of Pediatrics' Complaint

January 15, 1979

To: Phil Strong

From: Victor Alan

Re: Special Care Nursery Staffing Problems

Attached is Lydia Bailey's response to Dr. Ringo's latest memo.

I do not think that closing this unit at this time is in the interest of the East City community. I am asking Lydia Bailey to give us a follow-up report on training of nurses who work in the SCN and staffing in four weeks.

VA/nd

Att.

cc: Lisle Kent, M.D., President of the Medical Board
    Joseph Brocetti, President of the Board of Trustees
    Lydia Bailey, R.N., Director of Nursing

Attachment to Item 17

To: Victor Alan, CEO

From: Lydia Bailey, R.N.
         Director of Nursing

Date: January 11, 1979

Re: Letter from Dr. Ringo (1/8/79)

On Sunday, January 7, 1979, Sue Ellen Barnes, R.N. (a very qualified person for the unit) was scheduled to work 3–11 in the special care nursery. However, her mother called her in ill Sunday and we had a problem finding someone to cover the unit.

As you and the physicians are aware, it is difficult to find someone qualified for this area. We tried with no success to fill the slot with our qualified help who have adequate experience. Carol Soares, R.N., who was called and asked if she would cover the unit, said she would. When she arrived on duty, she felt a little unsure of herself and told the evening supervisor, who in turn called me at home. I gave her a few names to call to see if they could come in and give Mrs. Soares a hand. Not hearing anything to the contrary on Sunday evening, I assumed the situation was under control. On Monday, the supervisor told me she was unable to get anyone to come in and that Mrs. Soares was able to handle the situation. Therefore, she did not call me back.

It is true that Mrs. Soares did not have a six-week orientation to the special care nursery and I honestly don't believe anyone working in the unit has had six weeks' orientation before being placed on his/her own. But, once again, she is a qualified labor-delivery nurse and has worked before in the special care nursery and the regular nursery. I am not saying this makes her a qualified special care nursery nurse, merely that she is better than someone who has never worked there.

It is true that Mary White, R.N., has been in the special care nursery since the last experience which Dr. Ringo related to us, but with no ill effects. I've tried to put her as often as possible with experienced personnel for more orientation.

Mr. Alan, it is impossible for me to find the qualified help to run this unit. We have tried to cover this area with the most qualified people we have. I've hired an R.N. with experience for part-time 3–11 to start on February 12, 1979. At present, I do not have the staff to relieve someone for six weeks' day orientation to this area along with another six weeks on the shift they will work. I am very much aware of the fact that we are not able to provide the backup required to administer the quality of care we should be giving. Therefore, I agree with Dr. Ringo that this unit should be closed until we have the qualified help. I am not completely sure this is the answer, but I don't have the personnel interested in this area and I'm trying to recruit for same.

A problem I foresee in closing this area is that the personnel we have who are qualified will lose their skills and we will have to transport all these babies to the city. Another problem which comes to mind is who will maintain these babies after delivery until transfer to a city hospital if our labor-delivery nurses are not qualified to care for them. If they can't give emergency care to a baby in the delivery room, they will not have a baby to send to the special care nursery, let alone to the city.

I've talked to Violet Parple, R.N., and we are working on an orientation program with a skills list for each new employee. At present, I have full-time and part-time nurses on 7–3 and 3–11 who are qualified. My problems are the 11–7 shift and backup people. I am having difficulty finding people from our present staff who are interested in this area. I've discussed with Mrs. Parple bringing on days the present staff who have worked in the special care nursery. At this time she will evaluate and give more orientation if need be. I will rely on her judgment as to how much orientation these people need. Also, the present staff will have to fill out a skills list. This is going to take time; it can't be done overnight. As I said before, we're working on it.

Perhaps someone else has an idea on how to solve these problems. I will be meeting with the staff on January 18, 1979, and will ask them for their ideas. I will relate their ideas to you after this meeting.

Item 18: Memo from the Head of the Department of Laboratories to Community Hospital CEO Regarding Physician Authority, Staffing, and Cost in the Department

To: Victor Alan

From: Nicholas Poll, Laboratory

Subject: M.D. Authority, Staffing, and Cost in the
           Department of Laboratories

Your memo of January 30, subject as above, in my opinion actually should be divided into two sections, i.e.: (1) M.D. authority, and (2) staffing and cost in the laboratories.

It should be noted at this point that the ideas I express are my own. They are based upon observations here and at other hospitals, upon discussions with outsiders who are involved in the preparation of plans for the future in hospital care, and upon "leaked" legal and regulatory governmental programs under one or more of the "National Health Service" projections in the works and planned for activation in the not distant future.

It is quite possible—or rather, probable—that Alvin Castro, M.D., chief of pathology, will disagree with my thinking. Only the passage of time—which I estimate at not over three to five years from now—will prove which of us is right.

Your reference to M.D. authority I am sure has been an outgrowth of the complaint of one of our pathologists that, as a physician, he has been unable to obtain a clear definition of his authority in the laboratory in the time he has been here. It must be obvious that much of the situation has been left unsaid—and that with the impending departure of Bello, it is probably best left in that condition.

There is, however, a need to consider the matter of M.D. authority in the laboratories so that we avoid a repeat of the situation—at least to the maximum extent possible—with Bello's replacement. Here I can express my ideas.

A bit of history is in order. During the mid-1960s, the pathologists themselves realized that clinical laboratory work and administration had already become so complex—and indications were that they would become even more complex—that the mere possession of an M.D. degree, even with clinical pathology (laboratory) training, was no assurance that an individual could operate the clinical laboratories. Accordingly, the pathologists themselves created a new breed of management for the clinical laboratories—the laboratorian, or laboratory scientist, to take on the authority and responsibility of operating the laboratories. These laboratory scientists would have responsibility and authority in both professional and administrative operations. As the pathologists set the system up, a laboratory scientist could be either a physician clinical pathologist or a scientist with a doctoral degree in a related field. In either case, the laboratory scientist would have the specialized knowledge of laboratory investigation, analysis, instrumentation, administration, and so on. While a clinical pathologist physician or a chemist, microbiologist, and so forth could qualify and operate as a laboratory scientist, the mere possession of clinical pathology, chemistry, microbiology, or whatever training did not automatically qualify the individual to operate a clinical laboratory. Naturally, it was recognized that this new idea would lead to toes being stepped on and ruffled feathers, so new titles such as "technical director" (as opposed to "department head" or "director of laboratories") and "technical and administrative coordinator" were coined and placed in operation. In another hospital, my title of "clinical chemist" was changed to "laboratory scientist" in 1970.

Recently, the Joint Commission on Accreditation [of Hospitals] carried the idea one step further. The JCAH established requirements that IF A HOSPITAL OR OTHER LABORATORY PERFORMED SURGICAL PATHOLOGY STUDIES, THAT AREA OF THE LABORATORY *MUST BE* HEADED BY A PHYSICIAN. HOWEVER, THE *CLINICAL LABORATORIES* OF THE HOSPITAL COULD BE HEADED BY A PHYSICIAN PATHOLOGIST—WHETHER OR NOT TRAINED IN CLINICAL PATHOLOGY OR LABORATORY PATHOLOGY—OR BY A DOCTORAL SCIENTIST WHO WAS QUALIFIED UNDER THE LAWS OF THE STATE INVOLVED TO OPERATE A CLINICAL LABORATORY. In the latter case, a physician had to be available for consultation on medical matters, but the consultant need not be a member of the laboratory staff.

It might be noted that while the JCAH position does not greatly differ from that of the pathologists, the pathologists under their accreditation requirements have insisted that the department head or chairman be a physician pathologist.

This is where we stand at the present time. Now—how do I feel about the situation?

In my opinion, the authority within the laboratory must rest with the individual who has responsibility for the operation of the laboratory, and the measure of authority and responsibility must be equal. It should be obvious to any executive officer or administrator that, while he or she can establish basic operational policy, the authority to operate under that basic policy must rest with the individual who has the responsibility for operations. In our laboratory over the past few months, efforts have been made to retain authority for the pathologists, while passing responsibility to me. It is this factor which has led to some of the poor situations which exist.

Going further, I see no harm in subdividing authority, PROVIDED it is accompanied by subdivided responsibility. That the system will work was established to my satisfaction in Philadelphia, where I worked with three pathologists, each of whom—in my opinion—was a competent laboratory scientist. The four of us divided certain responsibilities—and the authority accompanying those responsibilities. This division did not prevent our working as a team—or from filling in for each other for vacations, time off, illness, and so on.

So far as our future is concerned after the departure of Lou Bello, I believe a decision must be made by you and Alvin Castro as to what you want in the new pathologist. Do you want a surgical pathologist with laboratory management experience? Do you want a clinical pathologist? Do you want a clinical pathologist with laboratory management experience? Do you want a department chairman—board certified in either or both surgical or clinical pathology—who will establish basic department policy and leave departmental authority and responsibility to others? These are not easy decisions, but I feel strongly that they will determine the shape of things to come.

In my own thinking, I would go for a clinical pathologist with laboratory management experience in every aspect of that management. I place this above the surgical pathologist because surgical pathology is only one of 11 sections of our laboratory. From a financial standpoint, it is the other ten sections of the laboratory which produce any potential profit for the laboratory and the hospital, and, today, laboratory management or direction cannot avoid involvement in the laboratory finances.

Again, so far as I am concerned: if we bring in a competent laboratory manager pathologist, who is willing to accept both authority and responsibility or to delegate responsibility and an equal amount of authority, I can and will work with him without problems. If we repeat the situation of the past few months, however, of attempting to divide or separate authority and responsibility, I see only a repeat of what has existed recently.

This has been a long, involved consideration of only one point in your memo, but your memo uses the word "detail," and the subject of authority can make or break what is to come. I hope the information presented will aid you in your own thinking.

The remaining questions you raise in your memo (staffing and cost) will depend upon the direction in which our laboratory is to go. It should be noted that these projections are not "long-range." We are talking, in my opinion, of things that will have to be done or established within the next three to five years. Either we will work out things we can live with and present them to third-party agencies, or the third-party agencies will tell us what we will do.

The following are the developmental possibilities for the Community Hospital laboratory (and probably for some of the other ancillary services we now provide).

1. Development of a laboratory to serve only the needs of Community Hospital.
2. Development of a laboratory to serve only the emergency needs of Community Hospital, with all other work being sent to outside laboratories, which would charge Community for the work performed.
3. Development of a laboratory to serve the needs of Community Hospital and to perform laboratory tests for other hospitals and institutions, charging the other hospitals or institutions for the work performed.
4. Establishment of a regional laboratory by a group of hospitals in the area, of which Community would be one, with the hospitals collectively owning the laboratory, paying the expenses of the laboratory according to their usage and sharing the profits of the laboratory according to their usage.
5. Development of emergency-only laboratories at Community and other area laboratories and utilization of a regional laboratory in the area operated by the pathologists of the hospitals but independently of the hospitals. Hospitals would pay for the work submitted, but any profits would accrue to the pathologists.

There are probably other possibilities available, but these seem to me to be the most likely. Each would create its own staffing and cost situations.

From the standpoint of the administration of the hospital, it is probable that #3 above is the best—and the one most likely to bring income and profit to the hospital. However, I do not believe we will be allowed to operate in this direction. It leads to competition between the hospitals for equipment, personnel, space, and so on, and I do not believe that the inevitable duplication of effort will be tolerated by third parties.

The system I see as offering the greatest possibilities is listed above as #4—a regional laboratory operated by a group of hospitals. This operation—in rented quarters at one of the hospitals or in its own quarters—would permit economical (high-volume) production, decreased competition for personnel, and elimination of equipment duplication. I am convinced that in the near future either we will submit such a plan of operation to regulatory or supervisory agencies or they will give us such a plan under which we will opertate—LIKE IT OR NOT.

Plan #5 above has just appeared in sight. A Canadian syndicate is attempting to set up such laboratories—operated and controlled by the pathologists. The United States manager of the program is Dr. Boring, who formerly was the director of the Center for Laboratory Medicine (CLM) (until the company was bought out by Damon and moved to

Texas). I have been told without confirmation that there is a group of pathologists in an area near here who have had some conversations with Boring.

In terms of staffing and cost, I think we have to consider:

1. Pathologist services,
2. Laboratory technicians and personnel services, and
3. Equipment cost.

In discussing pathology (specifically, surgical pathology) services, I enter an area where angels fear to tread. As part of my own thinking, I have tried for several years to obtain guidelines on what costs should be anticipated. Obviously the biggest single determining factor will be the surgical load of the laboratory. Unpublished (for obvious reasons) information from the College of American Pathologists gives as a guide that, with a general scope of surgical specimens, a single pathologist should be able to handle about 300 cases per month plus one autopsy per week. Unfortunately, the pathologist who gave me this information will deny having done so should the question be raised.

However, if we look at Community Hospital, which I would say has a general case load and type, we are seeing about 400+ surgical cases per month with an average of two autopsies per month. Based on the guideline given above, this would indicate that we would need two pathologists to carry our load. Review of our operations indicates that we probably could function within the guidelines.

There are, however, other factors which would have to be considered. If the pathologist is also involved to a significant extent with laboratory administration, there would be a marked reduction in the time available to him for surgical pathology, and additional pathologists might be needed. If the arrangements between the Hospital and the pathologist were via a professional association (PA), then the number of pathologists would be at the option of the PA, with any limiting factor available to the Hospital being the amount it would pay the PA.

It is not possible for me to project the cost of pathologist services based on need for the period ending March 1980, or for the period of three years after that date. It would appear that these are going to be subject to negotiation between the pathologist and the Hospital. I do feel, however, that, at some time in the not too distant future, percentage contracts will not be accepted by third-party agencies and that all hospital-based physicians will be salaried employees of the hospital.

In the area of laboratory technicians and personnel, the cost will depend upon (1) the coverage that must be provided (37½ to 40 hours per week or 168 hours per week or somewhere in between) and (2) the work load. Most expensive will be for a laboratory operating only for the Hospital. Least expensive will be for the regional laboratory, with its capability of operating three shifts a day, seven days a week. The profits being made by commercial laboratories which are able to operate in this fashion are proof of these statements.

Equipment costs over the next five years are equally difficult to project. The changing technology over this period may make almost all of our present-day equipment obsolete, and it is obvious that, as "new" technologies are presented, the cost of the newer instrumentation is heading for outer space. As an example, we purchased (leased) the Hemac Laser Hematology system 1½ years ago, when it was selling for $35,000. Laser measurements are one of the expanding technologies and will probably continue to expand markedly for the next 20 years. The second-generation Hemac is now being offered. It adds one more test to the seven previously measured—and the price tag is $85,000, 2½ times the price of the original system just two years ago. This is one reason why I have held back on requesting some equipment we can use right now—I haven't been able to learn what else "new" is just around the corner, what it is going to do, and what it will cost.

Yet we must think in terms of new equipment. By manual or manual-instrumented methods, a single tech can do about 15–25 tests per hour. Using automated instrumentation, his or her output can go to 60–300 tests per hour. The direction we must go in can be seen, if only we have the space and can pay for the automated equipment. Here, too, the benefit of regionalization can be seen. If we can collectively share in the cost of this equipment, and if we can collectively keep the equipment operating for more than a few hours in a day, we stand to come out way ahead.

I did not intend this reply to your memo to become a textbook, but, as I indicated to you, the memo throws me a curve—the ramifications are almost without limit.

I hope this information answers your memo—if not, please give me a call for specific details. If I disappear, you will know that Dr. Barnes* read a copy of the manuscript and I am sure he will disagree.

---

*Dr. Barnes is chief of pathology.

Item 19: Memo from Executive Secretary to Community Hospital CEO Regarding Patient Complaint About Quality of Care

To: Victor Alan, Chief Executive Officer

From: Sylvia Fliess, Executive Secretary

January 12, 1979

Mrs. Carocalla (362-0940) called me at 10 a.m. today and reported:

On January 3, she brought her 16-year-old daughter to the ER complaining of fever, stomach pains, headache. Dr. Bonus examined the girl *rectally* and diagnosed the condition as infected tubes, stating to daughter and mother that she had to have had sex to get the infected tubes. Girl denied this accusation and ran out of the hospital, having to be brought back by the nurse. Medication prescribed, which Mother purchased and administered, taking doctor's word of diagnosis. Mother still trusting her daughter, knowing that she does not date and is not allowed to go out at night, took the girl to Dr. Brise on January 11. Dr. Brise commented that infected tubes do come from having sex, BUT his examination revealed that the girl did not have an infection and was still a virgin. Diagnosis—flu.

Her other major complaint is that she does not feel that she should have to pay for the ER visit because her daughter was not diagnosed properly.

Item 20: Letter from the Chairman of Emergency Services to Community Hospital CEO Regarding Patient Complaint

January 17, 1979

To: Victor Alan

From: I. Bolles, M.D.

Re: Complaint from Mrs. Carocalla

I was already aware of this incident before Mrs. Carocalla complained, since one of our nurses had already informed me of the manner in which this young lady was diagnosed and the *improper* explanation given regarding the possible etiology of the disease she allegedly had.

I have spoken to Dr. Bonus regarding this situation, and he insists that he told the mother that sex was only one way to get infected tubes (although this is not the report I received from the nurse). I have informed Dr. Bonus that he should be more discreet in his approach to this problem, especially in view of the fact that a pelvic exam was not done, which would have confirmed her virginal state.

I can only ask that you express to Mrs. Carocalla our apologies regarding the error in diagnosis and inform her that we will do our best to prevent a similar reoccurrence.

Sources

I. Health Services Organizations

On his theory of organization: Parsons, Talcott. "Suggestions for a Sociological Approach to the Theory of Organizations." *Administrative Science Quarterly* 1 (1956):63–85, 224–39.

On the growth of the investor-owned hospital industry: American Hospital Association. *Hospital Statistics.* Chicago: American Hospital Association, 1978.

Federal HMO Legislation: U.S. Congress. P.L. 93-222, The HMO Act of 1973.

On the closure of New York City hospitals: Brecher, Charles and Roswick, Diana. "The City's Role in Health Care." In *Setting Municipal Priorities*, 1981, edited by Charles Brecher and Raymond D. Horton. New York: Russell Sage, 1980, p. 141.

On organizational adaptation: March, James G. "Footnotes to Organizational Change." *Administrative Science Quarterly* 26(1981):563–78.

A marketing bibliography: Robinson, Larry M. and Cooper, Philip D., *Health Care Marketing: An Annotated Bibliography*. Atlanta: U.S. Department of Health, Education, and Welfare, Center for Disease Control, March 1980.

On provider lobbying: Feldstein, Paul J. "The Political Environment of Regulation." In *Regulating Health Care*, edited by Arthur Levin. New York: The Academy of Political Science, 1980, pp. 6–21.

On teaching hospitals: Department of Teaching Hospitals, Association of American Medical Colleges. *Toward a More Contemporary Public Understanding of the Teaching Hospital.* Washington, D.C.: Association of American Medical Colleges, 1981.

II. Health Services Managers

On managerial functions: Longest, Beaufort B. *Management Practices for the Health Professional.* Reston, Va: Reston Publishing, 1980, pp. 45–50.

On managerial roles: Mintzberg, Henry. *The Nature of Managerial Work.* New York: Harper & Row, 1973, pp. 54–99.

On managerial activities: Allison, Robert F.; Dowling, William L.; and Munson, Fred C. "The Role of the Health Services Administrator and Implications for Education." In *Education for Health Administration*, Vol. 2. Ann Arbor: Health Administration Press, 1975, pp. 147–84.

On listening: Klion, Stanley R. and DeRusso, John J. Consulting Engagement Skills, mimeograph. Peat, Marwick, Mitchell & Co., 345 Park Ave., N.Y., N.Y. 10017.

On judgment: Brown, Ray. *Judgment in Administration.* New York: McGraw-Hill, 1966, pp. 14–21.

III. Managerial Contribution
to Effective Performance
in Health Services Organizations

On hospital performance standards: Griffith, John. *Measuring Hospital Performance, An Inquiry Book*. Chicago: Blue Cross and Blue Shield Association, © 1978, pp. 3–9. Reprinted with permission. All rights reserved.

On managing the public service institution: Drucker, Peter F. "Managing the Public Service Institution." *The Public Interest* 33(1973):46, 49.

On goals: Perrow, Charles. "Disintegrating Social Sciences." *Phi Delta Kappan* 63(1982):684–88.

On evaluating hospital CEO performance: Harvey, James D. "Evaluating the Performance of the Chief Executive Officer." *Hospital and Health Services Administration* 23(1978):5–21. Reprinted with permission.

On management evaluation: Pointer, Dennis D. and Strum, Dennis W. "A Framework for Management Assessment in Health Services Organizations" *Hospital and Health Services Administration* 26(1981):81–95. Reprinted with permission.

IV. Educating Health Services Managers

Cohen, Harold J. "Baccalaureate Education in Health Care Administration." In *A Future Agenda, Education for Health Administration*. Ann Arbor: Health Administration Press, 1977, pp. 57–69.

For information on programs in health and hospital administration and on the accreditation of these programs, contact the Association of University Programs in Health Administration. One DuPont Circle, Washington, D.C. 20036.

For information about programs in continuing education conducted by the American College of Hospital Administrators, write to them at 840 North Lake Shore Dr., Chicago, Ill. 60611. For Aspen Systems Corporation, 20010 Century Blvd., Germantown, Md. 20767.

V. Finding Your Niche

On jobs in health services management: Seixas, Suzanne. "A Glowing Future for Medical Managers." *Money* 9(September 1980):114–16.

Collins, Linda I. "Survey of Hospital Salaries." *Hospitals* 56(December 1, 1982);59–66.

For their surveys on graduates' starting salaries, contact Association of University Programs in Health Administration, One DuPont Circle, Washington, D.C. 20036.

On management contracts: Massachusetts Hospital Association. *Report of the MHA Task Force on Management Contracts*. Burlington, Mass.: Massachusetts Hospital Assocation, 1979.

On conflict of interest: *Resolution of Conflicts of Interest in Health Care Institutions*.

Chicago: American Hospital Association, copyright 1975. Reprinted with permission.

On the growth of for-profit health corporations: Relman, Arnold S. "The New Medical-Industrial Complex." *New England Journal of Medicine* 303 (1980):963–70.

On the professionalized bureaucracy and the divisionalized firm: Mintzberg, Henry. *The Structuring of Organizations.* Englewood Cliffs, N.J.: Prentice-Hall, 1979, pp. 466–67. Adapted by permission.

On multihospital management: Malm, Harry M. "Multi-Hospital Management: Analyzing an Example." In *Multi-Hospital Systems*, edited by Montague Brown and Barbara P. McCool, Germantown, Md.: Aspen Systems Corporation, 1980, pp. 301–324.

On multihospital management: Springate, David D. and McNeil, Melissa C. "Management Policies in Investor-Owned Hospitals." In ibid., pp. 324–42.

On multihospital management: Martin, Richard. Personal communication, 1982.

VI. Managing Yourself

On making executive decisions: Barnard, Chester I. *The Functions of the Executive.* Cambridge, Mass.: Harvard University Press, 1964, p. 194.

On time management: Webber, Ross A. *Time and Management.* New York: Van Nostrand Reinhold, 1972, pp. 60–93.

On interaction with subordinates: Ouchi, William G. *Theory Z.* Reading, Mass.: Addison-Wesley, 1981, pp. 127–28.

VII. Managing Your Team

On leadership: Burns, James MacGregor. *Leadership.* New York: Harper & Row, 1978, p. 19.

VIII. Working with Physicians

On conditional cooperation: Heclo, Hugh. *A Government of Strangers.* Washington, D.C.: The Brookings Institution, 1977, pp. 191–94.

On conflictive equilibrium: Saltman, Richard B. and Young, David W. "The Hospital Power Equilibrium: An Alternative View of the Cost Containment Dilemma." *Journal of Health Politics, Policy and Law.* 6(1981):408–410.

On organizational goals: Cyert, Richard M. and March, James G. *A Behavioral Theory of the Firm.* Englewood Cliffs, N.J.: Prentice-Hall, 1963, pp. 26–43.

On physician perspective: Freidson, Eliot. *Profession of Medicine.* New York: Dodd, Mead, 1972, pp. 158–84.

On physician mission as active intervention: Freidson, Eliot. ibid. pp. 252–57.

On colleague-dependent practice: Freidson, Eliot. ibid., p. 189.

On quality of care: Kessner, David M.; Snow, C.K.; and Singer, J. *Contrasts in Health Status*. Assessment of Medical Care for Children, Vol. 3. Washington, D.C.: National Academy of Sciences, 1974.

On quality of care: Breslow, Lester. "Quality and Cost Control: Medicine and Beyond." *Medical Care* 12 (February 1974):95–114.

On mental hospital admissions: Rosenhan, D.L. "On Being Sane in Insane Places." *Science* 179 (1973):250–58.

On overutilization: Ingelfinger, Franz J. "Arrogance." *New England Journal of Medicine* 303(1980):1507–11.

On medical cover-ups: Millman, Marcia. *The Unkindest Cut*. New York: Morrow, 1977, p. 93.

On the limits of medical knowledge: Freidson, Eliot. *Profession of Medicine*. New York: Dodd, Mead, 1972, pp. 335–58.

On physician fees as incentives: Blumberg, Mark S. "Physician Fees as Incentives." In *Proceedings of the Twenty-First Annual Symposium on Hospital Affairs*, edited by Roberta Baranowski. June 1979. Chicago: Graduate School of Business, University of Chicago, 1980, pp. 20–32.

On influence: Lindblom, Charles E. *Politics and Markets*. New York: Basic Books, 1977, pp. 17–64.

On medical records: *Accreditation Manual for Hospitals*. 1979 ed. Chicago: Joint Commission on Accreditation of Hospitals, 1978, pp. 76–77.

IX. Maxims for Managers

On aphorisms: Weick, Karl. *The Social Psychology of Organizing*. 2d ed. Reading, Mass.: Addison Wesley, 1979, p. 40.

Index

About the Author

ANTHONY R. KOVNER, MPA, Ph.D., is Professor and Director of the Graduate Program in Health Policy and Management, School of Public Administration, New York University. He is also Senior Program Consultant to The Robert Wood Johnson Foundation and serves as a member of the board of trustees at Lutheran Medical Center in Brooklyn, New York. He has previously been a health services manager in a nursing home, neighborhood health center, hospital (twice), and a group practice. Professor Kovner has served in a number of consultative capacities to hospitals, government, and educational institutions. He is co-author of *Health Services Management: A Book of Cases* (AUPHA Press, 1981) and *Health Services Management: Readings and Commentary* (Health Administration Press, 1983) with Duncan Neuhauser. He has also written numerous articles in several journals, including *Inquiry*, *Medical Care*, *Trustee*, *Hospital and Health Services Administration*, and *Hospitals*.